MW01290667

# Taking *Sexy* Back

## The Cure for the Sexual Blahs

Jean A. Campbell

authorHOUSE®

*AuthorHouse™*
*1663 Liberty Drive, Suite 200*
*Bloomington, IN 47403*
*www.authorhouse.com*
*Phone: 1-800-839-8640*

*First published by AuthorHouse   3/13/2009*

*ISBN: 978-1-4389-5284-0 (sc)*
*ISBN: 978-1-4389-5285-7 (hc)*

*Printed in the United States of America*
*Bloomington, Indiana*

*This book is printed on acid-free paper.*

This book is dedicated to my husband, Joe, whose curiosity and sense of wonder continue to infuse our relationship with passion and joy.

# Contents

# Acknowledgements

My heartfelt gratitude goes to my husband, Joe, who patiently endured and supported my first foray into book-writing and who didn't begrudge the dent this book ironically created in our own sex life during the final months of editing.

I have new appreciation and admiration for my incredible children, Leah and Brent, who courageously faced the daunting proposition of knowing more than most children ever want to know about their mother's sexuality. I am especially grateful for Leah's brilliant editing assistance during a tough year in law school.

I am deeply indebted to Bill O' Hanlon, my teacher, mentor, and inspiration for writing. This book may never have been written without his encouragement.

I am also filled with gratitude and appreciation for my original mentor and friend, David Steere, whose guidance started me on the path to sexual wholeness.

And, finally, to my unborn grandchild who represents the ultimate creative expression of sexuality, I anxiously await your arrival.

# Introduction

In 1971, I found my way to a small Quaker college in the Midwest. The war in Vietnam was still raging as was the revolution at home. I showed up on campus in my deerskin moccasins and old army jacket, ready to join up with other 18-year-old idealists in challenging the old order and ushering in the new. Campus living reflected the times – co-ed dorms, no rules, the smell of marijuana drifting down the halls. The sexual revolution was in full swing by then, and AIDS was still relatively unknown.

My sexual experience up to that point was limited to the boyfriend with whom I had happily relinquished my virginity at age 17. I felt worlds older after that coupling in the double-poster bed of my childhood and relished the secret life I had begun. But other than how to attract a partner who *wanted* to have sex with me, I didn't have a clue about the journey ahead. My instruction in the sexual realm prior to that first physical relationship had been covert and confusing. Once "it" happened, I knew the thrill of rebellion and the thrill of being desperately desired but precious little about my own sexuality. Though my boyfriend was more than happy to show me the ropes, his sexual learning was equally unhealthy and was driven by the frequency and force of his erections. He made every effort to satisfy me since that was a measure of his skill as a lover, but my focus was on pleasing him rather than discovering my own pleasure. I always answered 'yes' to his whispered question, "Did you come?" and I'd see a smug smile sneak across his face. Of course, I did discover some pleasure along the way, but I had bought my indoctrination as a sexual object, hook, line, and sinker. I faked not only orgasm but also endless enthusiasm for the sex that in actuality was only important to my partner. Why *would* sex be important to me? It had already served its primary function – it had won my lover's heart. That love ended when I went away to school, and my sexuality was once again up for grabs.

With the Pill eliminating the fear of pregnancy and puritanical sexual mores being part of the old order, there was little in my small college environment to inhibit "free love". Even when you wanted to say no, excuses required some self esteem and assertiveness which I lacked at 18, and "I'm not ready" sounded horribly old-fashioned.

Surrounded by male sexuality in warp drive and with an empty arsenal of sexual defenses, I began having unwanted sexual encounters that left me feeling empty and used. I couldn't say no. Ironically, the Christian upbringing that taught me to place a higher value on the needs of others collided with the breakdown of sexual rules, leaving me vulnerable to exploitation. Does it sound strange for me to say that my sexual willingness felt like a form of Christian giving? I had the means and the power to satisfy the sexual hunger of the poor young boys who sought relief in my body. It felt like I was sharing food with the starving or giving shelter to the homeless. The Patron Saint of Sexual Fulfillment. I was just practicing kindness – doing 'what Jesus would do' (if he were a female). And, of course, I was trying to get some of my needs met in the bargain, even though sex wasn't one of them.

I wanted to be liked, to be loved, to be wanted. I wanted to be a free spirit. But what I wanted most was a relationship. Unfortunately, my promiscuity got me none of those things. I still remember walking into World Civ and seeing the carefully averted eyes of the guy I'd had sex with the night before as he walked to the opposite side of the room and sat down.

And what of the boys who so casually took advantage of my sexual generosity? Did they ever feel empty afterward? Did they regret their pressure or false promises? Did their own sexual gratification trump the absence of mutuality and intimacy? If those questions seem strange, it's because we expect males to be sexual opportunists. Certainly, their sexual indoctrination did little to encourage restraint or discourage exploitation. But *was* there a price for the reckless indulgence of their sexual need?

My behavior, and that of my sexual partners, was at least partially a result of an absence of sexual wholeness. We were driven by sexual programming that defines women as sexual objects and men as sexual predators - programming that denies the full humanity and full sexual nature of both men and women. It's a setup for sexual dysfunction, power struggles, and eventually the loss of desire. Men and women pay a different price for bad sexual programming, but both pay a price.

My rocky introduction to sexual freedom in the early 70's started me on a search for sexual healing and sexual wholeness. Therapy helped me to incorporate my sexuality into a healthy sense of self. I stepped out of the role of sexual object and began to claim the power of my own sexual energy, thoughts, and feelings. After completing a degree in psychology and working for a time in the mental health field, I was drawn to the field of sex education. Following the sexual revolution, I saw little change in the unhealthy sexual identities of men and women, and I wanted to share a different vision of what it means to be a full sexual being.

I became a sex educator at Planned Parenthood and spoke to hundreds of groups about that vision. Hearing the stories of relationships awash in sexual struggles, I decided to work directly with the couples engaged in those struggles. Therefore, in 1986, I began a career as a marriage and family therapist. Through it all, I remained intrigued by our culture's curious approach to sex. This very powerful natural drive has been repressed, forbidden, distorted, exploited, manipulated, and less often, celebrated. No wonder we have so many examples of sex gone wrong.

As a marriage therapist, I have worked with far too many couples whose relationships have suffered because of sexual difficulties. High on the list of those difficulties is differences in desire. Of all the differences within a couple's relationship, it's one of the toughest ones to negotiate successfully. When couples find themselves at odds in their desire for sex, they often begin blaming, pouting, withdrawing, punishing, and accumulating resentment. It soon colors the entire relationship.

Within the last decade, there has been a significant increase in the number of my clients (and acquaintances) who report having very little, if any, sex drive. The stories I hear are plaintive, poignant, and strikingly similar:

> "I just don't have any sex drive anymore. Sex is still good whenever we get around to it, but if it weren't for Tom, I don't think we'd ever *get* around to it. Oh, maybe I'd miss it eventually, but it's fallen way down on my list of priorities. I never thought I'd be one of those women who'd make up excuses to avoid sex."

> "I retired last year and was looking forward to having more time with my wife, Sheila. My youngest left for college in the fall, and I had visions of Sheila and me chasing each other around our empty nest and making love in every room of the house. But now that I'm here, I just don't have that much interest in sex – and Sheila doesn't seem that interested either.

Maybe we've gotten so used to going without it that we don't think about it anymore. Maybe it's true what they say – 'if you don't use it, you lose it'."

"These days are a far cry from our early years together. I used to get tired of Kent's constant badgering for sex...now I could strip naked and dance around the living room and he'd be pissed off because I was blocking the TV. It's not that I've turned into a sex maniac or anything – it would just be nice to feel wanted once in a while. I wonder if it's him, or if I just don't turn him on anymore."

You get the picture. These stories are from people in their twenties and beyond, including the boomers who helped usher in the Sexual Revolution – who supposedly rewrote the sexual rules and celebrated 'free love'. A friend of mine who recently turned 50 remembers the exhilaration of being part of the generation that brought sex out of the closet:

"I guess the young have always felt like they were the first to discover sex, but with our generation, there really was a new discovery of sex. This was not the sex that our parents had – in the dark, under the sheets, missionary position. This was a wide open, buck naked, 'no holes barred' kind of sex that had never before been part of American culture. Not that no one before us had ever been sexually adventurous, but we were the first generation in this country to claim a right to it. We claimed a sexual freedom that shook things up and stood the old rules on their head.

It was a great time to be young."

We boomers may have taken sex out of the closet, but now it seems that an awful lot of people are shoving it back in. Who could have imagined that all that sexual energy that exploded back in the '70's would be replaced by apathy and a shutting down of sexual desire?

The more I heard about this sexual shut-down, the more I knew it was time for a second revolution – one driven not by hormones or rebellion against repression but by the genuine desire to claim passion and sexual wholeness. The first revolution didn't really change how we came to know ourselves as sexual beings – it simply gave us increased license to have sex. Unfortunately, permission does not create passion. This book grew out of my hope for a revolution that does create passion – that defines sexuality as something more than various body parts mixing it up – and that promotes a true integration of our sexuality. It's the only real answer to the epidemic of lost sexual desire. This book is about new paths to passion for all the 'grown-ups' whose sexual journeys are far from over.

# Chapter 1

## Why Banish the Blahs? The Power of Sex

I once heard a poignant story shared by a man whose marriage had been lacking closeness and intimacy for a long time. On their 25th anniversary, he decided to do everything he could to recapture the connection with his wife. He took her out for a romantic dinner at her favorite restaurant. Dinner was followed by a night of dancing to music provided by the same band that had played at their wedding reception. The evening seemed magical, and the husband saw a new light in his wife's eyes. They arrived home in the wee hours of the morning, still laughing like teenagers. Feeling like a newlywed, the man embraced his wife as they prepared to go to bed. Sensing his sexual interest, his wife's response to the loving embrace was less than enthusiastic as she pulled away and said curtly, "Now let's don't ruin a perfectly good evening!" The man confided that it was in that moment he knew he no longer wanted to stay in the marriage. It was too painful to want physical closeness with someone who wanted no part of it.

Jean A. Campbell

**What's Sex Got to Do With It?**

Sexuality is a key dimension of human existence. It's crucial to connection and happiness in a couple's relationship. Sadly, millions of men and women have allowed fading desire to determine the quality of their sexual lives. Without a sexual bond, relationships are less insulated from everyday stress and are more vulnerable to developing distance. Conflict often erupts over differences in desire which can further strain a partnership.

Studies estimate that low sexual desire affects over half of all women and at least a fourth of all men. Anecdotal evidence suggests those estimates may even be low. About 20% of married couples have sex less than once a month, and another 15% have sex less than twice a month. Those marriages may contain a high desire partner, but as is typically the case, it's the lower desire partner that determines sexual frequency. Half of married couples experience some kind of sexual dysfunction or dissatisfaction. But how important *is* sex in overall marital satisfaction? When sex is good, it adds 20-25% to contentment within a relationship, but even more compelling is what happens when you take sex *out* of the picture. Relationships take a hard hit when sex is bad, infrequent, or non-existent–affecting overall satisfaction by 75%. Obviously, the absence of sex is a major relationship drain. Is that just because the more highly-sexed partner is upset about the lack of action? Is it possible that sex is over-rated and over-sold? Unfortunately, that's the sentiment I've heard expressed by many people who simply don't have much of a sex drive.

## Why Do I Have to Change?

If you're happy hanging out in the sexual doldrums, why should you make the effort to move? Why can't your higher-desire partner just get over it? That would be one solution to the strain placed on relationships when sex is a source of conflict. There's even an organization for people who consider themselves not just low desire, but *no* desire. Founded by David Jay, who considers asexuality to be an orientation rather than a choice, the Asexual Visibility and Education Network now has more than 6,000 members. The organization is working to legitimize asexuality, and is probably a good arena for asexual people to hook up with a compatible partner.

Compatibility is essential. Unless both people in a relationship completely lack sexual interest, an asexual position dismisses an important need of a partner. When either partner has a significant need that is ignored within their relationship, resentment and distance usually follow. Asexuality also minimizes the individual benefits of experiencing oneself as a sexual being. Sexuality is a source of health and well-being both in relationships as well as in individual lives.

## What It's All About

Our sexuality is a vital source of energy. It's passion, engagement, and connection. Sex grounds us in our bodies and then allows us to transcend them in the moment of orgasm. It's part of the life force that fuels excitement and increases passion. The phrase "lust for life" conveys the intensity inherent in wanting and desire. It's no coincidence that lust is a word that describes both sexual desire and enthusiasm. Here's a sampling of definitions for lust:

As a noun:          Intense sexual desire or appetite
                    A passionate or overmastering desire or
                        craving
                    Ardent enthusiasm; zest; relish
                    Pleasure or delight
                    Desire; inclination; wish
                    Intense longing

And as a verb:      To have a yearning or desire

Wanting keeps us alive – and the wanting is for so much more than the physical act of sex. As Thomas Moore observes in *Dark Nights of the Soul:* "By bringing out your sensuality and vitality...sex can connect you to society and to the natural world...Sex involves precisely those things that are most important to the soul: love, curiosity, fantasy, desire, pleasure, intimacy, and sensation." We are innately attracted to the people who connect us to life. Just look at who it is that has the most sex appeal. It's hardly the sullen anorexic model on the runway who's about as appealing as a paper doll. The people we usually find sexy are those with energy, intensity, and passion – those who laugh often and are engaged in life.

I once had a colleague who inspired many sexual dreams in our years of working together. I was happily married and my colleague was gay, so for a long time I was puzzled by the dreams. Not that I minded them, but they made little sense to me at the time. Looking back now, I think the inspiration for the dreams came from my colleague's sexual energy and his engagement in life. He had a wonderful sense of humor, and the fact that he blushed easily and frequently didn't keep him from returning sexual banter. He was caring and compassionate and completely present in his interactions with people. What's sexier than that? At the going away party when he left the agency, I did a mock striptease for him to the tune of "I Can't Get No Satisfaction". But the truth is, I found our relationship more than satisfying, and still do. (The location of the videotape from that party remains a mystery.)

The syndicated columnist, Ellen Goodman observed, "We are…a culture that defines sexy as something seen rather than something felt." But sexy is far more than the images portrayed by Hollywood and Madison Avenue. Sexy is about feeling confident, being passionate about life, and being able to fully inhabit one's body, whatever shape or size. It's about claiming one's maleness or femaleness and becoming sexual beings rather than sexual 'doings'.

You can increase your 'sexiness quotient' by moving more awareness into your body and quieting those voices that question your worth. You can find something to get excited about every day even if it's just snagging a prime parking spot at the grocery store, and you can make it a daily goal to have at least one good belly laugh. Feeling good about yourself and being enthused about life may not land you on the cover of a magazine, but you'll definitely be sexy. Once you discover the close relationship between sex and a lust for life, you'll find it easier to experience yourself as a sexual being. Ultimately, sexy is how you go about making sex important when it no longer feels urgent. Nowhere is that more vital than in relationships.

## Sex and Relationships

### Is Sex Worth $50,000?

What kind of sexual connection do you share with your partner? Is there a sexual bond even when the sexual frequency is nothing to write home about? Do you still find your partner desirable and enjoy physical closeness with them? Most happy relationships are characterized by an enduring sexual connection long after the initial passion has faded. Chemistry and physical attraction color even the more mundane aspects of couple and family life. It helps hold a couple together through the ups and downs of life and helps them remember that they *are* a couple – not roommates or business partners or a parenting team. Sex is one of the most significant differences between your relationship with your partner and your relationships with everyone else. When sex is absent or problematic, both individual and couple happiness are affected.

There are a lot of different ideas about what goes into creating a happy life. I don't think many people would disagree, however, that the state of your primary relationship is a significant factor in your happiness. I recently ran across studies conducted at Dartmouth and the University of Warwick on the role of *sex* in happiness. The researchers concluded that "...increasing intercourse from once a month to once a week is equivalent to the amount of happiness generated by getting an additional $50,000 in income for the average American." I know a lot of people would argue with that conclusion and would gladly give up some sex for that amount of extra income, but it might be interesting to at least consider how much value sex adds to your life. If quadrupling the frequency of sex in your relationship wouldn't equate to $50,000 worth of happiness, how much would it be worth to you? How about to your partner? If sex isn't a big priority for you but it is to your partner, how would your partner's increased satisfaction affect your happiness?

Unfortunately, these aren't the questions a lot of couples are asking. Often sex is a source of *un*happiness in the life of a couple, and the only questions asked revolve around how to resolve sexual tension, desire differences, and resentment. Countless relationships have suffered casualties from battles between high desire and low desire partners. As differences in desire escalate, polarization often follows. The polarization creates positions or roles from which partners respond automatically – responses that are often contrary to their wants and needs.

Consider Ann and Dave's situation:

> Ann: "I think all Dave cares about is sex. I'm sick of the pressure, the crude remarks, the grabbing, the put-downs. I don't even want to kiss or touch Dave anymore because he'll think I'm ready to hop in the sack. Who wants to get up close and personal with someone who's pissed off and disappointed with you? I'm angry too – angry that I went through my dad's illness all alone and that Dave never pays attention to me until he wants sex. And the more pressure I feel, the angrier I get."

> Dave: "I can't even begin to understand not wanting to have sex with someone you love. When Ann makes sure she's always too busy for sex or turns away from me in disgust when I try to get something going, I feel unloved and unwanted – and not just in the bedroom. The more unwanted I feel, the more reassurance I need. But Ann thinks any time I want a hug or a kiss, I'll end up pushing for more. And to be honest, if it's been weeks since we've done anything, a kiss probably would make me want more. I know the pressure makes things worse, but if I don't push, then we never have sex."

Ann and Dave are each focused on what they're *not* getting from each other and end up responding in ways that perpetuate a negative relationship dynamic. Each shuts down emotionally after making the assumption that their needs are unimportant to the other.

## Sex – Not Just Getting Off

Actively identifying your partner's needs – both sexual and non-sexual – is critical. For the low desire partner, physical intimacy entails far more than physical interest. Ann may feel more receptive to sex if she feels supported and validated in the relationship. However, she may be missing the vital link between sex and the emotional intimacy she craves, just as Dave may be failing to recognize the inroad to sex found through meeting Ann's non-sexual needs.

There's often an assumption that the sexual interest of the high desire partner is strictly physical. Based on my conversations with high desire people, I've found that many non-physical needs are met through physical contact and that sexual overtures are often a bid for connection. The following are a few of the needs that people try to get met through sex:

- Closeness and Connection
- Fun
- Feeling Masculine/Feminine
- Making up/Reconnecting
- Stress Relief
- Expressing/Receiving Love
- Emotional Comfort
- Feeling Less Alone
- Feeling Attractive/Desirable

Jean A. Campbell

Individuals engage in sex for different purposes at different times and are often meeting multiple needs simultaneously. Because sex involves more than a physical release, sexual rejection is often interpreted as more than a rejection of the sex act, itself, but a rejection of the person as a lover and a partner.

If you're the higher desire partner in a relationship in which sex has become infrequent or non-existent, which of the following feelings have you had?

☐ Distant/Unconnected     ☐ Unwanted/Rejected
☐ Unattractive/Undesirable ☐ Physically Deprived
☐ Alone/Lonely            ☐ Less of a man/woman
☐ Frustrated              ☐ Bored, Shut down
☐ Touch Deprived          ☐ Resentful/Angry/Victimized
☐ Depressed/Hurt          ☐ Other _____

And if you are the lower desire partner in a low-sex relationship, which of the following feelings describe your experience?

☐ Distant/Unconnected     ☐ Wanted only for Sex
☐ Alone/Lonely            ☐ Less of a man/woman
☐ Angry/Victimized        ☐ Exhausted/Shut down
☐ Touch Deprived          ☐ Pressured/Resentful
☐ Disgusted               ☐ Cold/Numb
☐ Depressed               ☐ Other _____

When a couple with desire differences is stuck in a negative sexual dynamic, both are in pain, both feel victimized, and the relationship is put in jeopardy. A cycle of attack, blame, counter-attack, and withdrawal ensues. The way each partner responds to the other creates more distance, more hurt, more anger – and a slim chance of either getting their needs met, in *or* out of the sack. A new dynamic is needed – one in which both partners recognize the differences each bring to their physical relationship, and in which both are willing to meet those differences with understanding and acceptance.

Let's return to the story at the beginning of the chapter and imagine an ending that reflects this healthier dynamic. Remember the couple whose anniversary celebration ended on a sour note? This time, instead of pulling away, the wife warmly returns her husband's embrace. She shares her enjoyment of the evening and her renewed hope that they can begin finding their way back to one another. Though not yet ready for a sexual encounter, the wife asks her husband if he would be willing to hold her for awhile. He was hoping for more, but welcomes the chance for physical closeness. The couple falls asleep in the same spooning position they enjoyed in their early years together.

In the second ending, the wife is able to step out of her position of automatic resistance, and the husband responds not with disappointment, but with openness. Stepping out of habitual negativity and polarization is the first step toward resolving differences in desire.

It's not actually the differences in desire that exact a high toll on relationships but how those differences are managed.

## Low Desire – Not Just a 'Female Problem'

It's important to remember that men, as well as women, can find themselves on the low end of the desire equation. Millions of men just don't feel a lot of interest in sex. We don't hear as much about these men because they generally tend to keep quiet about their lack of desire. A man's sexuality is closely tied into his masculinity and his feelings about himself. Women less often associate their femininity and self esteem with their passion in the bedroom. Women talk freely with their friends about their lack of interest in sex and are typically met with understanding nods and knowing looks. Can you imagine a bunch of guys sitting around talking about how long it's been since they last got a hard-on? Men are reluctant to share anything that they think might reflect negatively on their penis or their sexual prowess. The secrecy is fed by the fear of judgment and the shame attached to feelings of sexual inadequacy. But I've heard the confessions of many men who stay up late watching television to avoid the sexual touch of their partners. They wonder what's happened to them and if they will ever feel lust and passion again. I've also heard from their partners – women who are craving affection, touch, and sex, and are struggling to understand their partner's absence of desire. So even though low sexual desire may not be an equal opportunity epidemic, there are plenty of victims on both sides of the gender divide.

## Sexual Awareness

Those with low desire can have a very rich sex life if they make sex a priority. Just as it isn't wise to wait until you feel a strong, spontaneous urge for exercise before heading to the gym, it isn't wise to leave your sexual life to the whim of natural desire. As a young person, your sexuality was defined by your desire or by the desire of your partner. As you age, however, it's important to expand your definition of what it means to be sexual. Your sexuality encompasses your sensual enjoyment of a cup of coffee on the deck or a massage from your partner, your ability to accept and enjoy your body, your innocent flirtation with the attractive waitress, and your joy in holding your children or grandchildren. The more you can stay in the moment and experience life with all of your senses, the more sexual you'll feel. You'll also increase your sexual awareness if you develop the ability to notice even the faintest stirring of sexual feelings. Building the equivalent of a searching image helps – selectively paying attention to sexual stimuli amidst the innumerable distractions of everyday life.

## Searching Image

My mom was incredible at spotting four-leaf clovers while going about her normal outside activities. Not searching down on her hands and knees in the grass – just, "Oh, there's a four-leaf clover" during a casual stroll around the block. Her ability to zone in on those tiny little clovers amidst a sea of green always amazed me. Now I know it was because she had a strong searching image of that clover.

A searching image narrows your focus and selectively screens out whatever isn't relevant. Someone forwarded me an email recently with a short video attached of two teams playing basketball. The instructions were to watch the video and count how many times the team in white uniforms passed the ball. After completing the task, you were asked if you saw the man in a gorilla suit who walked onto the court during the video. The majority of people who perform the counting task never see the gorilla. The counting task is the searching image, and it effectively keeps you from seeing other things happening on the court. Without a searching image for sex, you probably won't notice the internal and external cues that help maintain sexual interest. So if you're moving through your day counting the cars that fail to yield on the expressway while missing the sex gorilla, you may need to create a better searching image.

**Creating Desire**

Don't assume that desire is beyond your control. Just as you can have a desire to eat without being hungry, you can also have a desire for sex without physical arousal – or you can have a physical need that your body fails to signal. Are you one of

14

those people who don't feel hungry in the morning? That's a curious thing since the stomach is empty after a night of fasting. What's going on with that? If you're not hungry in the morning, it's because your stomach has given up on sending out a.m. hunger signals that have been consistently ignored. If you begin eating breakfast again on a regular basis, you'll notice the return of morning hunger pangs. A similar phenomenon occurs with sex. If you go long periods of time without sex, the body's sexual signals shut down. Resuming sexual activity brings desire back to life. Keep the action going regularly, and you may actually start to miss it when it's not happening. You may begin experiencing 'sex pangs'. It's another way of saying that desire often *follows* action rather than precedes it.

Sexual desire can be a willingness or a want to have sex. Focusing on the thought that sex will be an enjoyable experience and an opportunity to connect to your partner can increase desire. You have the ability to become a more sexual being and to make sex a joyful part of your life. The benefits extend far beyond the enrichment of your relationship.

## The Fountain of Youth

In a study conducted by David Weeks, a clinical neuropsychologist, 3500 men and women were observed through a one-way mirror by a panel of judges who then guessed the age of each subject. In those whose ages were underestimated by seven to twelve years, one of the strongest correlates was an active sex life. The most youthful looking group reported having sex at least three times a week compared to twice a week for the control group. Dr. Weeks suggests that when women have sex, the production of a human growth hormone is triggered that enhances a youthful appearance. If women put even half the time and energy into their sex lives as they put into efforts to preserve their youth, what a torrent of sexual energy would be released into the world!

Sex keeps you young. The 'youth' hormones – testosterone, estrogen, and DHEA – are higher in people who have regular sexual activity. Those hormones may no longer be raging, but they're a connection to a time when sex was new and adult life was just beginning. Those who have maintained their sexual vitality seem to defy our stereotypical portrayal of senior citizens as "dried up old prunes".

**Longer Life**

Not only does sex play a role in preserving youthful vitality and appearance, it may also impact actual longevity. Several studies have established that sexual activity is significant in extending lifespan. A long-term study in Ireland of a thousand men between the ages of 45 and 59 found that after 10 years, there was a direct correlation between sexual activity and longevity. The least sexually active men had a death rate that was twice as high as that of the most sexually active group even after accounting for many other differences. These Irish researchers also conducted a follow-up study in 2001 which found that men who had sex three or more times a week reduced their risk of having a heart attack or stroke by half. Pretty impressive medicine!

## Tension Release

During difficult times, sex can be a wonderful way to release tension. The relaxation response following orgasm can loosen tight muscles and help you step out of the over-identification with a problem. Just experiencing some moments not dominated by worrying thoughts can provide a welcome respite. Loving caresses and warm hugs reduce the level of cortisol in your body which produces a calming effect. Even stroking your cat or dog tends to lower blood pressure, so you can imagine what sex can do for you. Sex can certainly be shut down by stress overload, but sexual activity may also be one of the best stress management strategies you're not using.

## Mood Enhancement

The dopamine that's released during sex helps create not only pleasure, but a general sense of well-being. Semen even *contains* dopamine – along with estrogen, testosterone, serotonin, and norepinephrine – which means that women get an additional boost from this mix of feel-good chemicals. There's research demonstrating that women in monogamous relationships who have sex without condoms report lower levels of depression than a comparable group whose partners used condoms.

Studies indicate that the more often a person has sex, the happier they are. Now maybe happier people are just inclined to have more sex rather than the other way around. But what if all of the feel-good chemical and hormonal reactions that go on in your body when you have sex really do make you happier? It may be another reason to make sex a higher priority.

## Other Health Benefits

When was the last time your doctor encouraged you to include more sex in your life? Having regular sex should rank right up there with the standard health advice of eating right, exercising, and getting enough sleep. There are multiple health benefits associated with an active sex life. Sex reduces stress by lowering cortisol levels and improves immunity by increasing the number of infection-fighting cells and antibodies. Sex can provide certain kinds of pain relief and can also benefit reproductive health. Women are more likely to have regular menstrual cycles, and men increase their odds of having a healthy prostate gland if they engage in frequent sexual activity. Some studies have even shown that sex can have a preventive effect in prostate and breast cancer. Both sexes certainly benefit aerobically from sexual activity, as well. Not only are calories burned and heart rates elevated, but a number of muscles are given a workout and oxygen is pumped throughout the body.

And following that exertion and the release of sleep-inducing endorphins, there's the sexual benediction – a deep and restful sleep.

## Final Thoughts

So whether you're motivated to rev up your sex drive for the sake of your relationship or you want to plug into your sexuality for the enthusiasm, energy, and youthful vigor that it can spark, you and your partner will both reap the rewards. What else in a relationship offers more 'bang' for the buck?

When you're not plugged into your sexuality, you're not firing on all pistons. You're a sexual being, and by tuning into your sexuality, you can be healthier and happier. Low sexual desire is not a problem unless you allow it to cut you off from your sexual self. Desire is as much a decision as it is a feeling. That means you're in charge of deciding how to keep your sexual energy alive. Embarking on the journey to take sexy back begins with confronting your sexual programming and claiming the right to the sexual life you deserve.

## *Exercise*

If you're one of those people who just don't experience much natural desire, you've probably let sex fall pretty far down on your list of priorities.  Think about the benefits sex has to offer both you and your relationship.  Maybe you've thought of some benefits that weren't discussed in the chapter.  Which of these benefits will help motivate you to make sex a higher priority in your life?

☐ Closeness with my partner

☐ Less conflict with my partner

☐ Emotional comfort

☐ Fun

☐ Stress relief

☐ Staying young

☐ Improved health

☐ Exercise

☐ Longer life

☐ Other _____

How will you keep your motivation from being doused by the next deadline at work or the wallpapering project in the bathroom?  Make a plan for how to keep sex from being sidelined, e.g. "I'll make a weekly sex date with my partner and put it on my calendar."_____

_____

_____

# Chapter 2

## Screwed Over! Programming Problems

After a ten-hour shift at the hospital, Joanne rushed home and threw together a meal of frozen fish sticks and canned green beans for her and the kids. She hoped the video game sounds in the next room were just background noise for the kids working diligently on their math homework. Her husband, Jim, would be walking through the door at any minute from a weeklong business trip. The thought of getting up the energy for 'welcome home' sex was already overwhelming her. Luckily, when they crawled into bed later that night and turned out the lights, Jim was satisfied with a quick kiss before rolling over onto his side of the bed and going to sleep.

What's pulling the plug on the sex drive of couples all over America? From young couples in their twenties to the boomers who ushered in the Sexual Revolution, a spreading sexual malaise is catching people by surprise. When the spark of new love no longer generates erotic interest, many people are seeing their desire plummet. A few struggle to maintain some semblance of sexual interest, while others are content to exchange their silky underwear for holey briefs and granny panties. Those who have become indifferent about sex may find themselves at war with a partner who has desire to spare. Differences in desire often fuel sexual tension and negatively impact connection.

> Only one year into their marriage, the suggestive phone calls Leanne and Ethan once exchanged had been replaced by quick text message reminders to pick up a gallon of milk or the dry cleaning. Ethan's patience with long periods of abstinence was waning, and his snide comments about Leanne 'turning frigid' weren't helping matters any. Leanne wasn't even sure what that accusation really meant. If it meant just not caring about sex anymore, then maybe Ethan was right, but fighting about it all the time sure wasn't going to *make* her care.

Is sex really just the province of the very young and the very "in love"? If you're raising the white flag in the bedroom, you may feel at a loss to figure out, much less fix, the problem. This book is a guide through that confusion. Being 'screwed over' isn't a permanent affliction, and low desire isn't fatal to your sex life. Though our conditioning has created obstacles to healthy sexual functioning, there are solutions for the sexual challenges facing all of us. Before jumping into these solutions, it's important to first understand your own sexual programming and how it impacts your sexuality. The journey begins with how you first learned about sex.

## Sexual Programming

Your sexual learning began in the womb as you experienced the pleasure of sucking your thumb and touching your genitals. Because you'd not yet been told that exploring your body was naughty, you floated around in your protected little universe without guilt or shame. Unfortunately, that sexual freedom would soon be restrained as you began experiencing your sexuality in the outside world.

During early childhood, your parents gave you a sexual script. That script was written out of their own sexual conditioning and experience. Although the scripting probably contained some healthy elements, it may well have included significant hurt, shame, and inhibition, as well. Layered on top of the imprinting from your parents was a cultural script that contained mixed messages about sex: Sex is dirty. Sex is exciting. Sex is wrong before marriage. You're a loser if you're not having sex. Be sexy. Sexy is slutty.

This crazy-making indoctrination likely created confusion and uncertainty and may have set the stage for lifelong sexual difficulties.

> Jeff, a 31-year-old pharmacy assistant, came in to see me because he was unable to hold off ejaculating for more than a few seconds when he and his girlfriend had sex. Everything else in their sexual relationship had always been good, but he couldn't help feeling like a failure when it was all over so quickly. I asked about his early sexual learning, and he remembered his first real sexual feelings. "When I was 12 years old, I used to baby-sit for this family with 2

little kids. They had a magazine rack where *Playboys* were right out there along with *Reader's Digest* and *Life*. Swear to God! I couldn't believe it. Maybe I was sheltered, but it was the first time I'd ever seen anything like that. When the kids went to bed, I pored over those *Playboys* and got really turned on. That's when I first started masturbating… always listening for the sound of the car in the driveway and making sure I got the magazines back on the rack exactly like I found them before the parents walked in. I felt sneaky and dirty, but not bad enough to stop doing it. I just got it done fast so I wouldn't get caught. I started doing the same thing at home – in the shower, under the covers. Maybe I just got used to getting off as fast as I could. I don't know…now I just want to slow down and enjoy it, but I don't know how…"

For Jeff, *Playboys* embodied the message of open, free-wheeling sexuality. Unfortunately, everything else Jeff had absorbed about sex created a need for secrecy, followed by guilt and shame. His current sexual troubles are hardly surprising given his early sexual experiences.

## Gender Differences

To make matters more complicated, males and females receive very different social and sexual programming. Think back to grade school. What did you 'know' about boys? About girls? If you were to brainstorm a list of adjectives describing each gender – based on your early learning – you'd get a glimpse of the stereotypes that still reside somewhere within you. In the politically correct outside world, you've probably discarded many of those stereotypes. You may have even stretched way beyond the limits of that early conditioning in how you perceive yourself and the opposite sex. But once in a relationship, men and women often revert to stereotypical gender behavior with their partners. I'm not talking about who cuts the lawn and who changes the diapers as much as how power is shared, how couples communicate, who does the most accommodating, and who does the relationship-tending. Those dynamics have a direct bearing on intimacy and a couple's sexual relationship. Gender-specific sexual programming creates even more complexity. Both males and females receive covert and confusing messages about sex, but the gender differences in sexual learning create a divide that cheats both men and women of sexual wholeness.

## Femme Fatale

If you're a female, you probably grew up hearing more comments about your appearance than your achievements. It didn't take long for you to figure out what counted. You learned to use your looks to get what you wanted. Long before halter tops and low-rise jeans became part of your arsenal for attracting male attention, you smiled seductively, batted your eyes, and tossed your hair to get your way.

Coupled with cuteness was your growing ability to manipulate others using emotional and verbal skills. You acquired these skills at a much faster rate than your male peers because you learned to get your needs met indirectly. Discouraged from being aggressive, you used your feminine wiles to influence and persuade. With your bottom lip stuck out and a couple of tears running down your cheek, you could talk your dad into almost anything.

And what did you learn about your body aside from how to adorn it? Precious little, other than the need to keep your private parts private. You undoubtedly learned modesty early on. If you got caught playing with yourself or engaging in a game of doctor with a playmate, you were probably scolded with a tone of voice usually reserved for the dog that just peed on the carpet. You might not have understood why it was so bad, but you knew better than to ask questions. You'd already figured out intuitively that nobody talked about anything to do with *that* part of the body. You may not have stopped touching yourself, but you probably began feeling ashamed for doing so. Karen's experience illustrates the lingering impact of early shame-based learning about sexuality.

> "I don't know how I discovered masturbation, but I know I was young...probably 5 or 6 years old. I thought I was the only one in the world who did it or even knew about it...and it wasn't something I could exactly ask anyone about. I felt bad about doing it...but looking back...I'm not sure why. I just knew it was wrong. My family went to church a lot, and I started promising God I wouldn't do it anymore, but I'd always end up breaking the promise...Of course, now I know that it's normal and healthy, but I still feel a little guilty when I do it – and I wouldn't want anyone to know that I do it."

When you entered adolescence and became interested in boys, the emphasis on looks skyrocketed. You worried about being attractive enough and thin enough and big-breasted enough. Every pimple was a reason for panic, and a bad hair day had you begging your mom to let you stay home from school. Looking good and being liked were more important than grades, playing first chair flute in the orchestra, or making the varsity field hockey team.

When you were lucky enough to get a boy interested in you, things got a little more complicated. Whenever you were alone, he wanted to stick his tongue down your throat and grope your breasts. Sometimes that felt good and sometimes it didn't, but your own sexual responses took a back seat to managing the progression of his moves. You knew it was your job to set the limits because you'd heard often enough that boys were only out for one thing. The tricky part was figuring out how far to let them go and when. You constantly weighed the need to keep boys interested against the risks of going too far. When you finally went all the way, often under a great deal of pressure, you may have wondered what all the fuss was about. You probably experienced little pleasure in this adult rite of passage and struggled with the anxieties that followed. There was pregnancy and birth control to worry about, whether or not this guy really loved you or was just in it for the sex, whether you could keep your new sex life a secret from your parents, and whether you were going to hell.

Julie recounts her first time going 'all the way':

"It was the summer after my junior year – I guess I was 17 – and a bunch of us decided to go to the quarry. We waited until dark and climbed over this 6 foot fence that surrounded the place. One of the guys had swiped some

27

vodka from his parents and we sat around taking turns with the bottle. God, it was awful stuff! Pretty soon I found myself stripping off my clothes along with everyone else and feeling the shock of the icy water...then, the shock of arms grabbing me from behind and a slick body sliding against me. I'd never even kissed this guy before ...but it felt okay, and I let myself just go along with it. Before I knew it, he was leading me out of the water and behind a big rock close to the shore. Part of me knew exactly what was happening and couldn't believe I wasn't stopping it. Another part just seemed okay with doing whatever he wanted. I was still pretty drunk, but looking back, I don't blame it all on the booze. He was so sure of himself, so in charge ...I remember how raw it felt where he was pushing into me and then how quickly it was over. Waking up with a hangover the next day, I just kept hearing "I'm no longer a virgin" playing over and over in my head. I was scared...wondering if it was going to get around school and if I could be pregnant, but I also felt different...like I'd moved on to a new place."

Julie didn't plan to have sex. Like many women, she adopted a passive role in the face of her partner's aggressive and single-minded sexual pursuit. As we'll discuss in Chapter 4, women can challenge their early programming and move from being passive sexual objects to being the subject of their sex lives. There's an incredible release of passion in the shift from object to subject. It's a transition that opens up a whole new world of sexual possibilities.

### "Macho, Macho Man…"

If you're a male, you probably received very different messages than your female peers. You learned that it wasn't how you looked or how you felt that counted, but what you *did*. You were praised for competence and how effectively you acted upon the world. You also learned to stifle fear, sadness, and tenderness in your constant climb to the top of the heap. Performance was what counted, and competition for the *best* performance was the name of the game. Physical prowess was a measure of performance, and excelling in sports gained you big points on the masculinity scale.

You were implicitly invited to fully inhabit your action-oriented body and were proud of your penis. You and your private parts were well-acquainted since even peeing involved holding your apparatus. Modesty was less of an issue for you than for your female counterparts. Open urinals, group showers, and locker rooms gave you permission to accept your body – your whole body. Though you probably worried about 'measuring up' to other males in musculature and penis size, generally you were on good terms with your body, including your 'private parts'.

Adolescence was a treacherous time. As your voice deepened and erections popped up unexpectedly, you no longer felt in control of your body. Although sex was constantly on your mind, there was precious little outlet for all that sexual energy other than whacking off. You tried your damnedest to round the bases with the girls you dated, but it was usually more frustrating than successful. That didn't stop you from trying because even the girls who resisted ' your advances seemed to expect you to at least *try*. About the only prohibition you'd received about sex was not to get a girl pregnant. You didn't have to worry much about getting a bad reputation since you were only doing what guys were supposed to do – get it whenever, wherever, and with whomever they could. You can probably relate to Bob's experience.

> "I thought I was the only guy in the senior class who wasn't getting any. It's not that I wasn't interested – hell, if there'd been a masturbation Olympics, I would have earned the Gold – but every girl I dated just shut me down. Maybe I didn't have the right moves…or maybe I wasn't aggressive enough. It's not like there was anywhere to really learn that stuff, like Making Out 101. It was just trial and error….and for me it was mostly error."

There was little thought, and probably no discussion or instruction, about what sexuality really entailed. It was strictly a physical drive that dictated behavior designed to achieve physical satisfaction. In Chapter 5, we'll discuss the positive changes that occur when men move from a focus on sexual performance to sexuality that involves the whole self. When men begin to use both their heart and mind in sexual interactions, they free themselves from a lot of pressure and begin to experience sex in a much fuller way.

## The Sex Dance

Subjected to this faulty programming, girls grow into women who are much better at inspiring desire rather than *feeling* desire, and boys grow up to be men who are more comfortable relating to sex mechanically than relationally. Neither are whole sexual beings, and the dance between the sexes leaves a lot to be desired.

Playing the sexually passive role often results in many women feeling little desire once the romantic phase of their relationship begins winding down. They begin avoiding sex or simply going along with sex to get the closeness they crave. What's worse, they may start using sex as leverage to get other things they want from the relationship, like more help around the house, new dining room furniture, or greater emotional connection. And if they don't get what they want, the resentment starts to build. Being an object of desire is not exactly exciting when the house is overrun with laundry and a child is throwing up in the bathroom. Fran put it this way:

> "I guess it's a good thing Gary still wants me as much as he did when we first got together, but it grates on my very last nerve when I've finally gotten the kids settled, I'm finishing up the last of the pots and pans, and he starts humping me from behind. All I want to do at that point is sit down with a glass of wine and watch one of the shows piling up on the DVR. I don't even want to talk, much less get into the little bondage game he's whispering about. What I'd really like to do is cuff him to the bedpost and flee to the living room for some peace and quiet."

And what about men? Since their testosterone levels are 10-100 times that of women, their sex drive is not as vulnerable to the passage of time and the dwindling of romance. As they settle into a committed relationship, though, they may puzzle over what happened to the always-ready and eager-to-please sex partner they had in the beginning. They may even wonder if sex was simply a manipulative tactic to nail down a commitment. They now find themselves hinting, prodding, and pleading for the sex their partners once offered up with enthusiasm. As time goes on, their partner's sexual disinterest and avoidance builds resentment, and they begin pulling away. Eventually their own sexual desire, weighed down by work stress, fatigue, and disappointment with their partner, may start waning. Stretching out on the couch watching Seinfeld reruns might start sounding a lot more tempting than trying to get something going with a reluctant mate.

> Gary never thought he'd be one of those men who stopped caring about sex. Until the kids came along, he and Fran had sex almost every day – in bed, in the kitchen, in the shower, and on the couch during half-times. Then Justin was born, and Fran was exhausted all the time. "I knew a baby was going to change things. For a long time, I was okay if we managed to squeeze in a quickie once every week or so. It bothered me that Fran didn't seem to get into it anymore, but I kept thinking she just needed more time. When Justin was 2 years old, things got better for a little while. Looking back, I think it was all about Fran wanting another baby. As soon as she got pregnant, she went back to one excuse after another to avoid sex. I got tired of being pushed away and tired of being the only one who was really into it when she finally said yes. Maybe I'm the one making excuses now, but it just feels like too much work. It's not worth it."

Although low desire in both men and women is often exacerbated by fatigue, stress, and resentment, negative programming also creates sexual discomfort that diminishes desire.

## Squirming

A client recently explained to me that her low sex drive was a result of a childhood in which anything having to do with sex was "hush-hush and nasty". Welcome to the childhood of most people over the age of 40. Negative indoctrination can put a significant crimp in your comfort level with sexuality and make you squirm at the mere thought of poking and prodding into the whole dirty business.

If you're a squirmer, you probably don't think much about sex at all. You're not in touch with your own sexual feelings, you're uncomfortable with your body, you most likely try to have just enough sex to keep your partner from walking out, and it's difficult, when you do have sex, to relax enough to get anywhere close to orgasm. Actually, I'm shocked (but pleased) that you're reading this book! Maybe you've decided to find out, once and for all, what the rest of the world seems to know about sex that you don't – or maybe you're being pressured into reading this book by your higher desire partner. Whatever the reason, your willingness to explore the sexual domain is the first step in challenging your negative sexual programming.

## Facing Fear

After deciding that you're going to do something about your programming, you then have to be willing to step out of your comfort zone. No one likes being outside of their comfort zone, even a little bit, because it makes them, well – uncomfortable. As soon as you're outside of that zone, anxiety and fear will try to bully and intimidate you into returning to your place of comfort. However, you are not fully engaged in life if you allow fear to be in charge of your decision-making. Unless you're willing to stand up to fear in the same way you would stand up to any other bully, you'll be unlikely to discover the sexual joy that lies waiting on the other side of your discomfort. You have to decide that sex is important enough to warrant feeling the fear and moving right on through it. Just as I wouldn't want you to miss out on claiming a multi-million dollar lottery prize because of your fear of publicity, I don't want you to miss out on all of the delight that sex has to offer just because it's easier and safer to stay where you are.

> Sarah came in to see me because she finally "got" how important it was for her husband to have a partner who enjoyed being intimate. Ironically, her recognition came only after her husband had finally given up on ever having the sexual relationship he wanted to have with her. He had pressured, ranted, and pouted, but eventually he'd reached a point of acceptance. When he decided that he loved Sarah enough to stay with her despite their very infrequent and passionless sex, Sarah was touched and saddened. Though she had never had any interest in sex, she decided she wanted to do whatever she could to enjoy lovemaking with her husband.

This commitment to change put Sarah way out of her comfort zone. However, the discomfort Sarah felt was trumped by her desire to please her partner and improve their relationship. If her husband was willing to stick with her regardless of her sexual disinterest, she was willing to work on getting more interested. The potential benefit outweighed the risk.

## Baby Steps

If you're out of your comfort zone in the sexual arena, it's important to go slowly and take baby steps in the direction of sexual freedom. Before doing anything differently with your partner, you need to start with yourself. Begin by tuning into the messages and voices inside of your head that make you feel embarrassed, ashamed, or 'bad' for exploring your sexuality. Identify who the voices belong to – your mother? Your father? Your Sunday school teacher? Decide whether the messages reflect your current values and belief system or whether they're simply imbedded in the sedimentary layers of your formative years. If the messages aren't in sync with your present-day wisdom and values, then challenge them. Talk back to them. Notice the absence of logic or reasoning in the messages. Imagine that you have successfully reprogrammed yourself and are completely comfortable with your sexuality. How would you then respond to the destructive messages you've internalized about sex? Do some journaling. It's helpful to write a dialogue between the old voices and the new voice you are claiming.

> Sarah had a hard time challenging her internal tapes about sex. The old messages that kept looping through her brain felt like the 'truth'. I asked her to think about what kind of messages she wanted to pass on to her daughter about sex. She was then able to connect to a wiser part of herself

and identified a very different set of 'truths'. This wisdom allowed her to successfully challenge the old tapes.

## More Baby Steps

Once you've stood up to your fear and put your mind in a different place, then you can slowly – very slowly – begin introducing some of the strategies described in later chapters. Do some reading about sexuality, tune into your senses, become more aware of your body, and explore non-sexual touch with your partner. You don't need to rush. If something you try feels too uncomfortable, go back to the previous step and stay there for awhile before moving on. If you're trying new things with your partner, ask for time and patience. Continue to challenge any shaming messages that come up.

> Because Sarah had never had an orgasm, I asked her to read *Becoming Orgasmic*, by Julia R. Heiman and Joseph Lopiccolo. The graphic descriptions of the female genitalia and the methods suggested for stimulation of the genitalia were difficult for Sarah to even read. I suggested that when her discomfort became too intense that she stop, take 3 deep breaths, and repeat some calming statements. Then she could either go back to reading or give herself a break until another day. Sarah stayed at the thinking and reading stage for several months before she was ready to take the next step.

## Trauma

Sometimes sexual shame and guilt is a result of early sexual experiences that were hurtful or scary. Someone may have exposed himself to you on your way to school; you may have played 'doctor' with a playmate and been caught by an irate parent; you may have been touched or fondled by an uncle or a grandparent; you may have been date raped as a teenager; or you may have been sexually abused for years by an older sibling or a parent.

The statistics on sexual abuse vary, but it's estimated that roughly one in four girls and one in six boys experience some form of sexual abuse before the age of 18. There may well be over 40 million survivors of childhood sexual abuse in this country. It's reasonable to assume that without help, many victims of sexual abuse struggle to create healthy sexual relationships in their adult lives. If enjoying your sexuality is difficult because of past abuse, it's important to seek help from an experienced therapist. Together, you can achieve the reprogramming necessary to enjoy a rich and healthy sexual life.

## Final Thoughts

With scripting and programming that reduce sexuality to a sexual act performed by animalistic men on grudgingly indulgent women, it's actually surprising that joyful, mutual lovemaking exists at all. Your beliefs form the infrastructure of your script and are powerful in shaping your experience of the world. What you believe about sex in general, and what you believe more specifically about your own sexuality and that of your partner, has a great impact on your sexual life. If the programming you received created a script tainted by shame and negativity, your sex life is going to suffer. Thankfully, despite the resiliency of programming, it isn't permanent. When you're aware of operating out of negative sexual beliefs, you can begin challenging them. It's never too late to adopt a belief system that promises new possibilities for your sexual enjoyment. Sorting out the lies from the truth and doing some re-writes on your script are the first steps to healing your sexual wounds. By refusing to remain a victim of bad programming, you're already well on your way to taking sexy back.

## *Exercise*

Think about your own sexual learning and what kind of sexual programming you received. Use the following questions as a starting point for discovering and challenging your sexual script. By sharing your answers with your partner, you can reduce shame and bring greater compassion and understanding to your sexual relationship with one another.

1. When you were growing up, how was nudity handled in your family?_____

_____

_____

2. What kind of privacy did family members have in the bathroom and when dressing?_____

_____

_____

3. Did you shower or bathe with your mom or dad?

_____

Were you bathed with a sibling? _____

If you bathed with other family members, how old were you when it stopped? _____

4. How did your parents refer to the private parts of your body?_____

_____

What were your first words for the private parts of your body? _____

_____

5. When did you first discover that touching your private parts felt good?_____

_____

_____

When did you first masturbate to orgasm? _____
_____

How did you feel about masturbating? _____
_____

6.  Did you ever engage in sex play with another child?\_\_\_\_\_
_____
_____
_____

Were you ever discovered by an adult in sex play with another child? _____
_____

How did the adult react? How did you feel? _____
_____
_____

7.  Did any adult ever touch you sexually when you were a child?_____
_____
_____
_____

8.  Did you ever witness anything or hear anything sexual?\_\_
_____
_____
_____

Could you hear your parents having sex? _____

9.  Did you ever look at pornography as a child?_____
_____

How old were you when you were first exposed to pornography? _____

10. What did you learn about sex from your religious training?

_____

_____

_____

11. What did your parents tell you about sex?_____

_____

_____

_____

12. Did your parents talk about sex openly in the family? Tell sexual jokes?_____

_____

_____

_____

13. How did you first learn about intercourse?_____

_____

_____

_____

14. How did you learn about menstruation, wet dreams, masturbation, etc.?_____

_____

_____

_____

15. During your teenage years, what did you learn about pregnancy, sexually transmitted diseases, rape, sexual abuse?

_____

_____

_____

16. Who or what was your primary source of information about sex?_____

_____

_____

_____

# Chapter 3

## From Powerlessness to Passion

There was probably a time in a galaxy far, far away, when you and your partner couldn't keep your hands off each other. You carefully plotted and planned sexual liaisons and hungrily anticipated feeling flesh against flesh. Or you didn't plan, and the back seat of the car, an elevator, or the kitchen table sufficed. But chances are, as you started preparing Power Points, changing diapers, and cleaning the gutters, sex became a low priority. Unfortunately, having *any* kind of fun with your partner became a low priority.

I routinely ask a couple in the first therapy session about the last time they went on a date. As the couple looks at each other searchingly, the response typically goes something like this:

> "We went to that wedding a couple of weeks ago.... and there was that company picnic...but maybe that doesn't actually count as a 'date'...we did go to see "Spiderman" when it first came out, but it was the first one, so it's been awhile..."

It's not at all unusual for couples to go months without having any special time together. Everything else takes priority. During courtship, we make time for weekend canoe trips – even while facing a Monday morning deadline. But once the romantic phase of the relationship draws to a close, it seems we decide that fun is no longer important, and we settle into the serious business of scrubbing the toilets, getting our teeth cleaned, and making sure the cats get to the vet.

Do you expect your car to change its own oil or your clothes to jump in the washer? Even the small things that are important in our daily life require regular maintenance. And we certainly wouldn't expect our children, our friendships, or our jobs to run on automatic pilot without falling apart over time. But in our primary relationship, we operate with the false assumption that 'all you need is love' (to quote the Beatles). The *feeling* of love, however, is as transient and unreliable as an octogenarian's erections. The only love that's lasting and dependable is love that's nurtured and actively tended. It requires commitment, dedication, and the ability to tolerate disgusting noises and Lifetime movie marathons. The payoff of lasting love is a partner who sits by your side in the hospital, at the movies, and throughout your niece's entire three-hour ballet recital.

If you're guilty of relationship neglect and have allowed distance to grow between you and your partner, your sex life probably sucks – and not in a good way. The absence of sex is both a cause and effect of distance. Bridging that distance is one of the ways to get back into the game, and planning more fun is a good place to start.

## Reclaiming Fun

Do you ever watch couples in a restaurant and guess which ones are married? They're often the ones staring silently into space, more focused on their linguini than on each other. Simply spending time together isn't always a path to connection. Going to dinner and a movie can be a pleasant way to spend an evening, but it's not quite the same as skinny dipping or swing dancing. In the early days of a relationship, there's more intensity and passion brought to the table – and not just for lovemaking. Walking on a golf course at midnight, picnics in the park followed by a turn on the swings, making love in the woods, overnight trips to see your favorite band, riding the Ferris wheel and feeding each other cotton candy – see the difference? Romance induces playfulness, silliness, and a wonderful child-like ability to be fully in the moment. Though it may not come as easily as in the beginning, you can be more deliberate about keeping fun in your life and in your relationship. Not that there's anything wrong with crashing at home on a Friday night to watch Casablanca – but if one of you is checking email and the other is folding clothes, you're unlikely to create much connection or passion. The clothes and the email can wait until morning.

When my husband and I met, we both worked full-time and were each custodial parents of young children. Time was at a premium. My job at a non-profit agency paid poorly so money was also in short supply. With such scant resources, a courtship proved to be a tight fit, but we still managed to squeeze in an incredible amount of fun and excitement. Of course, it helped that our idea of fun included midnight trips to White Castle and browsing through Target, and exciting was anything that involved just the two of us. There wasn't a time before or since when I've had as much on my plate, and yet for three years, we managed it all and still found time for each other. Understand that by managed, I mean beanie weenies or fish sticks for dinner, sometimes getting one of the kids to ball practice more than a few minutes late, and rarely getting more than 6 hours of sleep. I've often kidded my husband that the reason I accepted his proposal was that I couldn't take any more phone calls that lasted until 1:00 a.m.! However, like most couples who are newly in love, we fought hard for couple time even during the busiest and most demanding period of our lives. I wish I could say we've been just as consistent in nurturing our bond throughout our twenty-three years of marriage, but occasionally we've allowed ourselves to be distracted by crises and the demands of everyday life. During the challenging years of raising three teenagers, the loss of parents, the stress of moves, job changes, and surgeries, it was sometimes easy to forget *why* we were an 'us', and even easier to neglect that 'us'. It was during times like these when I'd tell my husband we needed a 24-hour getaway. I needed reassurance that I wasn't out of my mind when I said, "I do". And if money was in short supply, I'd mentally calculate the cost of two divorce attorneys and decide that our getaway was a bargain.

## Battling Fatigue

A female client recently told me about a nice lunch she'd shared with her husband after they'd snuck out of work to get an early start on the weekend. On their way home, he asked, "You know what I wanna do when we get home?" Thinking about her latest purchase from Victoria's Secret, she was about to respond encouragingly when he yawned and said, "I wanna nap until dinner. It's been ages since I've had a nice long nap." So much for her dessert.

When love is new, we're a lot more motivated to make time and energy for each other – and for a post-lunch dessert. I know I had a list of 15 babysitters and sometimes made 11 phone calls just to arrange for a night out. But when you settle into real life, the motivation fades and intimate time together seems less important. You may feel so worn down that crashing in front of the TV in your sweats sounds like a better option than heading to bed a little early for some one-on-one time. If you're frequently tired and sex comes in a very distant second to sleep – or TV – on your list of priorities, it's important to address the sources of your fatigue. Stress, multiple demands, and a long to-do list are standard fare in most people's lives. Those raising young children may wonder if there will ever come a day when sexual interest and romance compete successfully with the constant fatigue that's so debilitating during the early years of child-rearing. Caught up in parenting, jobs, and household responsibilities, a couple can become little more than business partners just chugging their way through each day's agenda. Add in poker night, book club, choir practice, and kid sleepovers, and it's no surprise that operating under sleep deprivation is the norm in our society.

In *Just Do It*, a book by Douglas Brown that details his experiment with having sex for 101 straight days, fatigue was one of the biggest obstacles he and his wife faced. They often collapsed into bed at the end of the day desiring nothing more than a good night's sleep. But they learned something about fatigue as they pursued their sexual marathon – they discovered that it soon dissipated when it was actively challenged. During the experiment, the husband remarked to his wife, "If you stand up to the fatigue, it falls to pieces...it's a cheap bully." His wife reflected, "Exhaustion is a cheap bully. That's *awesome*...that knowledge alone is worth this experiment." Basically, this couple with full-time jobs and two young children just ignored the fatigue and began touching and caressing each other until the desire showed up. The desire then banished the fatigue. It's similar to when you force yourself to go for a walk after dinner when what you really want to do is nap on the couch. You return from the walk with a renewed energy that carries you throughout the rest of the evening. Getting enough sleep is the ideal in preserving energy for sex, but it's helpful to remember that you can also decide how much power you're willing to relinquish to fatigue. Asking for help is another method of preserving energy.

## Ask for Help

If you're doing more than your fair share at home, it's time to re-evaluate the distribution of labor. Tell your partner it's tough to be an eager bed buddy when you're exhausted and filled with resentment over carrying too much of the load. Anger contributes greatly to stress and fatigue and can suck the life right out of the warm, fuzzy feelings for your partner. Be specific about asking for help, and don't get hung up on the belief that your partner should anticipate your needs. Many women hold a strange belief that their partners should think, feel, and act as they would in the same circumstances and then get pissed off when they don't. They get stuck in a negative refrain: "Why should I have to *ask* him to run the sweeper? He can see the piles of dog hair!" Worrying about what's right or fair keeps you from doing what works.

Another barrier to getting help from a reluctant mate is the fear of a negative or angry response to requests. Sometimes even a loud sigh from a partner who's been asked to clean out the fireplace can be disheartening enough for a woman to conclude, "It's just easier to do it myself." Melissa was one of those women who had a really hard time asking for help.

"I don't know why I've always had such a problem asking for what I need. Maybe I thought I should be able to do it all, or maybe I expected Walt to know what I needed and just provide it. I know I've been afraid of him getting mad if I asked him to do something he didn't want to do. I don't handle anger well – at least other people's anger. Of course, I was feeling angry a lot. I knew I needed to do something different, so I finally got up the nerve to tell Walt I needed his help around the house. Granted, I started small. I asked him if he would load the dishwasher and put the food away after dinner. He didn't seem to mind at all. I couldn't believe it was that simple. I know he probably won't always be so agreeable, but it's worth taking the chance."

An alternative to constantly asking for help with routine chores is to sit down with your partner and develop a plan for taking care of the household, including the who, what, and when for each task. Or set aside a regular time for doing weekly chores together, like a couple of hours on Saturday mornings. Be willing for your partner to do tasks differently and imperfectly. It is *not* earth shattering for towels to be folded in half rather than in thirds (though I'm quite sure the latter is the proper method!), and though my husband will never remember to use the coupons I give him for the grocery store, the savings sacrificed are a small price to pay for some freed-up hours.

Hiring some help is a third option. Though it might seem to be an unaffordable luxury, the savings in wear and tear on your relationship could be worth every penny invested. You could always forego the kitchen remodeling project that would probably just have you at each other's throats anyway.

The main objective is to keep household chores from becoming a source of repetitive conflict. If you and your partner are stuck in a power struggle over who does what or who does more, the power struggle is going to spill into the bedroom – and chores have no place in your sex life. After doing your best to negotiate an equitable division of labor, acknowledge that it's never going to be perfectly equal and let it go. There will always be something your partner does or doesn't do that you find irritating or frustrating. If you have little sexual interest, you can use those frustrations as a way to avoid sex. Instead of addressing the problems in your sexual relationship, you can manufacture grievances to justify your avoidance. You may have legitimate complaints about your partner's behavior, but don't use the dirty dishes or the un-mowed lawn as an excuse for shutting down your love life.

## Making Sex a Priority

You're going to go through times in your life that take busyness to a whole new level – one of you is in law school, you just had a baby, one of your parents is in the hospital, or you're working 18-hour days to meet a project deadline. These are times when sex just isn't going to fit nicely into the picture. But life happens, and unfortunately, sex is often the first thing to go when something has to give. Ironically, the support derived from the physical comfort and closeness of sex is often critical in managing the stress of finals, 2:00 a.m. feedings, hospital vigils, or project jitters. Sex doesn't have to be at the top of the list during these crazy times, but it needs to be a high enough priority that it doesn't fall *off* the list.

Even in ordinary times, relationships can be cheated of time and energy that's diverted to individual commitments and activities. The activities may be worthwhile – sitting on community boards, serving as a Boy Scout leader, helping a friend paint his house, teaching a class at church, babysitting for your grandchildren – but need to be evaluated in light of the impact on your primary relationship. I've heard many clients complain bitterly about a partner who devotes huge amounts of time to church, volunteer work, or community activities and has little left over for them. Don's story is typical.

> "I think it's great Ruth has a lot of interests and is involved in the community, but now she's gone 3 or 4 nights a week. She's in two book clubs, a gardening club, and is president of her investment group. She's also on the board of two different organizations. I could handle her being gone several nights a week if she didn't come home totally wiped out. She doesn't even want to get a bite to eat, much less do anything after we go to bed. If she's that tired, why can't she drop a few of her activities? The truth is, I think she'd rather do those things than spend time with me."

It's healthy for individuals to have interests and involvements they pursue independently. There are legitimate needs that a partner simply can't meet, and having multiple resources for need fulfillment takes some pressure off the primary relationship. So how do you know when your activities become a liability to your relationship rather than an asset? Take an honest inventory and assess whether your involvements energize you and give you more to bring back to your relationship or whether they deplete you and diminish your ability to be a giving partner. How many activities have you taken on because you just weren't able to say no? To what degree are your activities avoidance, and to what extent are you trying to get needs met outside the relationship that could be met by your partner? It's often easier to look to outside sources for fulfillment if your attempts to get your needs met with your partner have ended in frustration. But taking the easy way out creates more distance and less incentive to meet and resolve the problems head-on. You can't make sex a priority if you don't first make your partner a priority.

**Nurturing Desire**

Janice was amazed by the turnaround in her relationship with Ben once she began initiating some of their sexual encounters.

> "I was sick of Ben's constant badgering for sex, and he was always pissed off when I wasn't interested.

All the pressure was just too much. At first I felt guilty, and so I just started shutting down. I talked to my sister about it, but instead of taking my side, she got on my case for not taking any responsibility for the situation. That irritated me, but after some consideration, I decided to take her up on her offer to loan me her slutty nurse costume. I actually had fun thinking about turning the tables on Ben and planning a little surprise check-up. It had been over a year since I'd initiated any action and, I have to say, I didn't need a stethoscope to tell Ben's vitals were a little over the top when I started his examination. Taking more initiative has really turned our sex life around. We still only have sex about once a week, but that seems to be enough for Ben now that he knows he doesn't have to push so hard to get anything to happen. Maybe it also helps that he feels like I'm interested."

The low desire person typically puts all of the responsibility on their partner to initiate whatever sexual encounters take place, and then waits for their partner to push the right buttons and create the magic that will turn them on. Hardly fair, is it? Though ostensibly in a passive role, the low desire partner holds a great deal of power. There's a lot of control in getting to decide if, when, and how sex takes place. A couple's sexual dynamic can come to resemble a game of cat and mouse. Just as the power of the cat is often over-estimated relative to its prey, a disproportionate degree of power may be attributed to the more aggressive partner in a relationship. Both partners can end up feeling like victims when control in the sexual relationship isn't shared.

To share control, the lower desire person not only needs to make sex a priority but needs to actively nurture passion – to be intentional about building tiny flickers of interest into the desire to *feel desire*. A low desire person may never have spontaneous sexual feelings or urges, but having little or no natural craving for sex doesn't mean that sex can't be enjoyed. Once "in the mood", a low desire person can take just as much pleasure from sex as their higher desire partner, even though the 'mood' may not strike until sex is well underway. For a sexual relationship to thrive in the absence of physical desire, there has to be an openness to experiencing the pleasure that will *create* desire. Focusing on enjoyable sexual memories and the benefits of a close physical relationship can foster greater interest in maintaining an active sex life.

In taking a more active sexual role, you can pick the times and circumstances for sex that work best for you. Maybe you have more energy for sex on a weekend afternoon than late on a weekday night. Maybe you're more likely to get in the mood if you first take a warm bath and slow down your racing thoughts. Maybe you need time to think some sexy thoughts, fantasize, read some erotica, or watch a steamy movie. Or, maybe you need to first feel emotionally close to your partner through spending some non-sexual time together. When you pick the time and the setting for sex, you're much more likely to be a giving and a responsive partner. You'll also avoid the dilemma of either refusing your partner's interest or forcing yourself to respond. Your investment in closeness is a great gift and allows your partner to feel wanted and desired.

Another reason for both partners to share the responsibility for their sexual relationship is that over time, desire levels shift and change. Medical conditions, grief, loss of a job, depression, and menopause are only a few of the factors that may cause a high desire person to lose a lot of their sexual drive. If the high desire person has assumed total responsibility for initiating sex in the relationship, their loss of desire may precipitate a complete sexual void.

A client of mine, Ted, always wanted sex more frequently than his wife, Janet. Despite their differences in desire, they had a pretty decent relationship and an enjoyable, although infrequent, sex life. When Ted began to experience depression and started on an antidepressant, he felt a noticeable decline in desire. But unlike many men, he felt more relief than concern because his sex drive became more in sync with Janet's – which was okay for awhile. Ted and Janet enjoyed sex a couple of times a month, and that frequency suited both of them. But when Ted began having increased difficulty reaching orgasm, intercourse ended up being 20-30 minutes of frustration rather than pleasure, which in turn caused Ted to avoid sex. When sex just stopped altogether, more and more distance began creeping into the relationship. At that point, Ted brought

Janet in with him for a joint session. When they made the commitment to therapy, it had been six months since they had been physically intimate. Janet had not particularly missed the sex, but she longed for the closeness they'd once shared. In the session, Janet volunteered to share responsibility with Ted for restoring their physical relationship. They also agreed to explore alternate ways of being intimate. Both recognized the importance of keeping sex in their marriage.

**Staying in Balance**

Ever notice what happens to sex when you're sick or physically worn down? How about when you're emotionally distraught? Or when you're mentally distracted by a fight with your best friend? Do you feel like getting it on when you're feeling empty or questioning whether your life has any meaning? Your sexuality is not merely anatomical or mechanical. It's sensitive to everything you experience and is inextricably intertwined in all of the dimensions of your life. When you neglect your physical, emotional, intellectual, relational, or spiritual health, your sexuality is going to take a hit. What you're looking for is balance, and it begins with you. Only by practicing good self care can you achieve that balance and then be capable of giving abundantly to your relationship. A balanced self generates greater passion for life and energizes your sexuality.

## Emotional Self Care

Our emotions convey important information. They let us know we're alive and how we're faring at each particular moment. Anger lets us know that something is wrong or that we have a need that is going unmet. Sadness is usually a signal that we've lost something important to us and are grieving for that loss. Fear helps us prepare for a threat to our safety and prevents us from taking unwise risks. Finally, joy is our cue to celebrate life's blessings. The challenge is how to *have* our emotions without *being* our emotions. Because we use 'to be' verbs to describe our feelings – "I *am* sad", "I *am* angry" – it's easy to step inside a bubble of emotion and forget that we're much more than our boredom or our jealousy or our crankiness. Once inside the bubble, it's tough to keep a healthy perspective and even tougher to do any real problem-solving. How likely are you to think clearly when you come home early from a weekend getaway to find beer bottles on the front lawn, the house trashed, and your teenage son passed out on the living room floor?

Anger is a particularly difficult emotion. The first stage of anger can be so overwhelming that it may demand a physical response just to release the adrenalin surging through your body. Hopefully, that physical response doesn't involve throwing your son out on the lawn with the beer bottles, but you may need to scream into a pillow, take a brisk walk to the nearest Baskin and Robbins, or furiously run the vacuum cleaner to release your frustration. Then, after your heart has stopped pounding and you can take some deep breaths, focus on your thoughts. You're probably telling yourself stories that amplify your victimization: "How could he take advantage of us like that? After all we've done for him..." or "He's completely irresponsible. He doesn't care about anybody but himself!" Although in the above example there may be some truth to those characterizations, these are the same kind of stories we generate when we're angry with our partner. "That damn fantasy football is more important to him than I am. He doesn't care about my needs at all..." Try considering some alternative stories that incorporate the perspective of the other person. For example, "He's usually a good kid. Maybe things got out of hand before he could stop it..." Or in regard to the fantasy football, "I know he works hard and needs some down time. Maybe we just have different ways of unwinding..." These kinder, gentler stories will help defuse your anger and move you closer to problem-solving.

Ultimately, engaging your rational mind is the best strategy for recovering from emotional imbalance. You may still *have* the feeling, but you're less likely to be defined by it. Simply allowing feelings to run their course can result in long periods in which you're unavailable to your partner. It's normal for sexuality to be eclipsed by strong emotions such as anger, sadness, or fear, but you have some control over how long those feelings stick around. It's really about learning to soothe yourself. Self-soothing involves rediscovering your center when you've been thrown off-balance. It means stabilizing your emotions and not over-reacting to others, especially your partner.

A relationship offers many opportunities to practice self-soothing. When your partner forgets your anniversary, expects you to cook the day you get home from the hospital, or just insists that history will prove George W. Bush was a great president, it's easy to lose your equilibrium. When you can take a deep breath, engage your mind, and become comfortable in your body, you can stay connected to your partner even when tension surfaces.

We've been talking about the range of emotions that all of us experience in the normal course of living. However, if sadness becomes depression or worry becomes debilitating anxiety, it may not be possible for you to get in charge of these emotions by yourself. If depression or anxiety is compromising your quality of life, seek help from a therapist. Depression and anxiety are both very treatable, but left untreated can affect every part of your life. You cannot begin to generate sexual interest if it's a struggle just to get through the day.

**Physical Self Care**

When you're in pain, out of shape, sick, tired, or sick of being tired, your partner is more likely to drive you crazy than drive you wild with desire. Though we've all heard it many times before, physical self care requires that you eat right, exercise, and get enough sleep. If you're not taking care of your body, it's simply not going to function properly. Maintaining good physical health is essential to keeping your sexuality in good working order. When your health is compromised, the body's energy is used up combating whatever is impaired, and your libido suffers.

Eating a healthy diet enhances your overall health, but paying attention to what you eat can also benefit your sex drive. Eating too many refined carbohydrates triggers the release of excess insulin which, in turn, creates a deficit of sex hormones. And though we've all been cautioned to watch our fat intake, eating too little fat can actually decrease your libido. Your body needs fats in its production of testosterone, estrogen, and other hormones. The best diet includes protein, fresh fruits and vegetables, complex carbohydrates, and some good fats – from olive oil, flaxseed oil, canola oil, and nuts – thrown into the mix.

Everyone knows that exercise helps maintain a healthy weight, but it does far more than keeps a check on your love handles. Exercise helps manage stress, anxiety, and depression – all of which can interfere with sexual desire. Several studies indicate that women who exercise are more sexually responsive. That may be due to endorphins that are released during exercise, or it could be that women who work out tend to be in better shape and have a healthier self image. Either way, women who exercise tend to be more in tune with their bodies and may be more responsive to physical cues, as well. Regular exercise, for both sexes, increases rather than decreases energy, which is always a boost to the libido.

Though alcohol has long been viewed as an aphrodisiac of sorts, alcohol is actually a depressant and can interfere with sexual functioning. Though a few glasses of wine may aid relaxation and soften the mood, the softening effect may extend further than you'd like! Even when sex isn't on the agenda, excessive alcohol consumption typically creates isolation and emotional distance. Far too often, I hear complaints about the partner who comes home from work, has several drinks, and falls asleep on the couch. This isn't exactly the recipe for a 'night of love'. Smoking also impairs sexual functioning. Because smoking constricts the blood vessels and affects the flow of blood to the penis, it's a major cause of impotence. Thailand even posts sex warnings on cigarette packs! The U.S. might do well to incorporate that caution in their anti-smoking campaign.

Along with taking care of your health, it's important to work on body acceptance and body awareness. If you walk around disconnected from your body and your senses, you're unlikely to experience sexual desire even if you're in great shape. It's just as important to be sure you're *enjoying* your body. Your body is an incredible source of pleasure and sensual delight. If you're not relishing the smell and taste of freshly baked bread, delighting in the sound of your child's laughter, or luxuriating in the warmth of a fireplace on a chilly night, you're neglecting your body. Develop an appreciation for your body and all that it does for you. Make sure you're also using your whole body when you make love. Genitally-focused sex is limited and overly goal-oriented. The body contains literally hundreds of erogenous zones for enhancing pleasure and increasing eroticism, and the five senses are vital components of sexual response. Physical self care isn't about harsh regimens or masochistic denial. It's about maximizing your physical health in order to more fully embrace all that life has to offer. Sex is one of those offerings.

## Intellectual Self Care

For many people, life has taken on a grim sameness – get up, go to work, come home, eat dinner, read the paper, watch television, go to bed. The routine varies some on the weekend, but is still largely filled with repetitive chores and errands. To keep your mind alert and engaged, it's vital to shake things up periodically.

Your mind craves new input and challenges. Novelty is energizing – it releases endorphins that make you feel good and spark your sexual interest. Whether it's eating at a new ethnic restaurant, training together for your first mini-marathon, trying out a new sexual position, or sleeping out on the deck on that first warm summer evening – doing something to break up the energy-sapping monotony of everyday routines helps rev up both a passion for living and for your partner.

The brain also receives a welcome jolt when you engage in behavior that's slightly risky. When you push yourself to do something with your partner that's just a little scary, it releases dopamine in the brain that enhances both pleasure and bonding. It's up to you to evaluate the risks, but bungee-jumping, skiing, or making love in a secluded outdoor spot might add more than excitement to your relationship.

I met my husband in a single's group which was made up of divorced men and women in their 30's and 40's ready to have a good time. One woman in the group was an avid white water rafter who regularly organized trips to the major white water rivers within a 200-300 mile radius of Louisville. My husband had already been down several rivers when I met him, and being newly in love made me more courageous than usual. So the first months of our courtship included several terrifying and exciting trips down Class IV and V rapids and one less-than-graceful fall out of the raft. I'm not sure how much that influenced our bonding, but it definitely created a lot of fun, thrills, and good memories.

If high-risk adventure isn't your style, just try learning something new together. Take up salsa lessons, sign up for a foreign language class, or learn how to sail. My husband and I have been taking ballroom dancing lessons with some friends for the last two years. You'll never see us on Dancing with the Stars, but it's been challenging and different. More recently, I made the leap from reading by the stream in which my husband was fly fishing to letting him give me some casting lessons. I don't know how frequently I'll use the waders and hip boots I found under the Christmas tree last year, but I've enjoyed sharing more intimately in one of my husband's great passions.

Ongoing mental stimulation and learning – with your partner and on your own – will help you stay energized and keep your mind sharp. Whether it's doing the daily crossword puzzle, reading before bed each night, taking on a new challenge at work, or learning Tai Chi, intellectual gymnastics keep your mind from going to mush and help you stay engaged in life. It also makes you a more interesting and lively partner.

**Relational Self Care**

The relational dimension includes not only your primary relationship but your relationships with family, friends, and coworkers, as well. It's pretty easy to see the correlation between the quality of your primary relationship and the quality of your sex life. Although the impact may be less evident, your sexuality is also affected by your relationships with others.

The people in your life can support and sustain you, or they can tear you down and drain your energy. Sometimes the same people do both. As social creatures, we depend on others to share our sorrows, celebrate our successes, hold our confidences, give us encouragement, keep us grounded, and help us when we need assistance. But what if the people in your life – including family – are of the critical, demanding, energy-zapping variety? You may need to set limits on the amount of time you spend around negative people, even those who are family. You can try gently challenging the negativity, e.g. "Mom, I know you're concerned about me, but whenever you bring up my weight, it just makes me want to run home and wolf down a gallon of ice cream. What I really need is to feel like you accept me whether I lose weight or not." That may work, and it may not, but it's worth a try. If the negative influences in your life are friends, it may be time to cultivate some new friendships. Take a class, join a club, or get involved in the local food bank – anything that will allow you to interact with people who are improving themselves or working to improve the lives of others. One of the lives improved could be your own.

The nature of your regular interactions with others and the overall quality of your relationships will either enhance your life or make your life more difficult. With so many demands depleting you, it's vital that you have a rich support network of satisfying relationships to help fill you back up. The more you are filled up – emotionally, physically, intellectually, and relationally – the more you are energized, and the more charge you'll have in your sexual battery.

## Spiritual Self Care

The last dimension to consider in battling sexual inertia and claiming sexual wholeness is spirituality. Does that surprise you? For those of you still battling sexual guilt and shame from religious indoctrination, sex – at least *good* sex – and spirituality may seem mutually exclusive. But spirituality and religion are not synonymous. Religion may play a significant role in your spiritual world, but the essence of spirituality is how you define meaning in your life. Without meaning, you're at a loss to make sense out of the world. Spirituality also supplies you with a compass of sorts to guide your life choices. Neglecting your spiritual life puts you at risk for depression and a sense of emptiness that can carry over into your relationships and into your sexual life. It is purpose and meaning that energize and motivate, help you overcome adversity, and bring depth to the connection with your partner. When you're in touch with the sacred within you and within your partner, sex isn't exploitive or hurtful. Sex becomes a truly mutual experience of giving and receiving and ceases to be appearance-focused or performance-based.

If your spiritual life seems lacking, some exploration may be in order. Read books about spirituality, different religious traditions, or philosophy. Take a meditation class or visit a variety of churches, synagogues, or temples. Spending time in the company of those who share your beliefs helps strengthen and mobilize the principles guiding your life, as well. Do some journaling about your beliefs and what's important to you. Spend time in nature, which can be both grounding and uplifting. Talk to spiritual leaders in your community whom you respect and find out the basis of their belief system. If there is someone you know and admire who doesn't use religion as their spiritual reference point, ask them how they define meaning in their life. One of the people I admire most is unerringly ethical, charitable, and loving – and a professed atheist. She's a committed environmentalist and derives meaning from her efforts to save the planet from humankind's exploitive consumption of resources. Although you'd be unlikely to ever hear her speak of spirituality, you wouldn't need to spend much time in her company to know that she's a person with purpose, values, and depth.

Defining and nurturing your spirituality will help you to stay centered and focused on what is important. Incorporating the spiritual dimension into your sexuality will bring in the divine aspect of your capacity for feeling ecstasy and giving joy. As Philip Sudo says in *Zen Sex*:

> "At its best, sex takes us back to the beginning, transcending mere fulfillment of of our animal desires to reveal our inherent divinity as Creators; it becomes a spiritual endeavor, as profound as any religious rite...All it takes to be a good Zen lover is a giving heart, and the awareness of the life force coursing through our bodies."

**Final Thoughts**

Attending to the intellectual, emotional, relational, physical, and spiritual dimensions of your life keeps you balanced, energized, and whole. By learning to fill yourself up in each of these five areas, you'll be happier, healthier, and sexier. There's tremendous power in passion. Excitement infuses your life with joy and intensity and shakes up the status quo in your relationship. When you reclaim fun and nurture desire, fatigue no longer shuts down your sex life. Sex becomes a *source* of energy and replenishment and an indispensable element of the abundant life you deserve.

## *Exercise*

What is dragging you down and putting a damper on your sex life?

Which of the five dimensions of your life – intellectual, physical, emotional, relational, or spiritual – need some attention to get you more in balance?

Take a moment to consider what changes you could make in the following areas and jot down a plan of action for enhancing your equilibrium.

**Fun**

☐ My partner and I make fun important
☐ My partner and I have high-energy, laugh-out-loud time together at least twice a month
☐ My partner and I know how to be silly and child-like
☐ I put time and energy into planning fun times with my partner

Plan of Action _____

_____

_____

_____

**Fighting Fatigue**

☐ I regularly get 7-8 hours of sleep each night
☐ I am able to say no to requests that push me past reasonable limits
☐ I ask for help from my partner and my children
☐ I prioritize my tasks and make sure there's some "me" time most every day.

Plan of Action _____

_____

_____

_____

## Nurturing Passion and Making Sex a Priority

☐ I am intentional about keeping sex on my to-do list
☐ I make sure that my outside involvements don't leave me too exhausted for sex
☐ I actively encourage sexual thoughts and take the time to get myself in the mood rather than expecting my partner to do all the work
☐ I initiate sexual activity with my partner

Plan of Action _____

_____

_____

_____

## Emotional Self Care

☐ I have good stress-management skills
☐ I generally stay on top of depression and anxiety and seek help when I need it
☐ I journal or talk to someone when I'm upset
☐ I am able to manage anger without bottling it up

Plan of Action _____

_____

_____

_____

## Physical Self Care

☐ I get some form of exercise on a regular basis
☐ I eat a healthy diet and maintain a comfortable weight
☐ I get enough rest
☐ I stay away from tobacco and limit my alcohol intake

Plan of Action _____

_____

_____

_____

## Intellectual Self Care

- ☐ I vary my routine periodically to keep things interesting
- ☐ I have an outlet for my creativity
- ☐ I look for new and different things to do with my partner
- ☐ I challenge my brain daily by reading, doing crossword puzzles or learning something new

Plan of Action _____

_____

_____

_____

## Relational Self Care

- ☐ I have a good network of supportive and nurturing people in my life
- ☐ I limit the time I spend with people who bring me down
- ☐ I make time in my schedule for friends and family
- ☐ I turn to my support system in times of need and ask for their help

Plan of Action _____

_____

_____

_____

## Spiritual Self Care

- ☐ I have a sense of purpose and meaning in my life
- ☐ I spend time with others who share my sense of purpose
- ☐ I feel centered and in sync with the universe
- ☐ I have a regular spiritual practice that helps me to stay centered

Plan of Action _____

_____

_____

_____

# Chapter 4

## The Rebirth of Venus:
## From Sex Object to Sex Subject

I think I was about 13 years old when it really hit me that I had something guys wanted. Not that I was hot stuff – I was a skinny, awkward adolescent who wore glasses and dressed in clothes my mother whipped up on her ancient Singer sewing machine. But I had long legs and budding breasts, and I reveled in the once-overs and whistles of approval from random horny men on the street. I never really thought much about sex, but I got the distinct impression that whatever it was that guys were looking for, I had it. Of course, the 'it' was little more than being an anatomically correct female, but I liked getting that approval – like getting a gold star for being a girl. To increase the interest we were arousing, my best friend and I would sometimes pad our 32AA bras with tissue and strut our stuff down a busy street just to see how many cat calls we could get. I have to admit, it was pretty exhilarating.

## The Four A's

Females learn very early on that their sexuality is a powerful tool for capturing male attention. Starting as young as 10 or 11 years old, girls parade around in halter tops, short shorts, and skin tight jeans, and are thrilled with the stares and flirtation they attract. There's not much thought about what those stares mean, like whether a boy's interest may be limited to the physical package, but there's an acute awareness of sexual power. The power is directed toward being noticed and getting a boy interested.

So what happens after a guy is interested? Whether it's a 16-year-old girl or a 30-year- old woman, a similar game unfolds. She must keep him interested while, at the same time, try to enforce whatever physical limits she decides are appropriate. And, of course, what's appropriate changes with the times, the culture, and the peer group. Recently, there's been an upsurge in the number of young teenage girls engaging in casual oral sex with multiple partners. What's in it for the girls other than the four A's - acceptance, approval, affection, and attention? These needs are primary motivators for female sexual behavior. In an effort to fulfill these needs, females begin focusing solely on being desirable.

By early adolescence, girls already begin to recognize how much of their *value* lies in being an object of desire. Cindy, a 15-year-old girl, put it this way:

"If you're a girl, it's all about how you look. Guys

worry about how they look too, but they can get away with a whole lot more. Girls have to look 'hot' if they want any attention from guys. You have to be sexy, but not slutty. It's the same with how far you go with a guy – you have to put out some or you're not really sexy, but then if you go too far and with too many guys, you get a bad reputation. Like, there was this guy I'd just started hanging out with who wanted me to give him head. I know a lot of girls are doing it, and a lot of guys just seem to expect it. But I worry about something showing up on My Space –like somebody calling me a 'ho' Sometimes it feels really messed up."

With so much focus on arousing male desire, even at very early ages, a female's own desire becomes secondary. Because her sexual feelings often fail to create a pressing physical need, they are relatively easy to ignore. Females who are sexually aggressive are typically driven less by sexual desire and more by the need to *be* desired. Female desire often doesn't begin to play a major role in her sexual behavior until it's turned on by the neurotransmitters that start firing when she falls in love. Infatuation is a powerful aphrodisiac for a female, and it sparks a new awareness of her sexuality.

## Love Potion #9

The sexual feelings experienced when a woman falls in love are a result of elevated dopamine and testosterone levels. Under the influence of these chemicals, even a woman with normally low sexual desire will often feel and act like a person with high desire. Unfortunately, when the romantic phase of the relationship eventually comes to an end and the chemical love potion begins to wane, so does a lot of female sexual interest. Females may still derive pleasure and fulfillment from sexual encounters initiated by their mate, but they less frequently provide the enticement that characterized the early stages of the relationship. They may even start to experience their partner's sexual desire as an irritating or draining demand and may begin meeting sexual advances with avoidance or resistance.

And what's it like for the partner of this siren turned sleeper? He may feel tricked and blindsided by the disappearing interest from his previously passionate partner. He may struggle to make sense of the transformation and take it very personally. Applying his own logic and worldview, he assumes that his partner's vanishing desire is the result of diminishing attraction. Bill, a 50-year-old man whose wife frequently finds excuses to avoid having sex, expressed his hurt and confusion.

> "When I first started dating Sara, she was hot! I couldn't believe I'd found a woman who liked doing it as much as I did. She'd talk dirty to me and we even acted out some fantasies. She was a total turn-on for me. Then, about a year after we got married, she just seemed to lose interest. She was always doing something with her daughter – who's 25 – or was too tired or just not in the mood. I don't know if

there's someone else or if she's not in love with me anymore."

The question Bill is really asking is, "If she still loves me and still finds me desirable, then why wouldn't she want to have sex?"

## From Object to Subject

Bill's question is legitimate. He may not understand his partner's different experience of sexuality, but she likely minimizes the value of sex in their relationship. A woman's sexual response is less elemental than a man's and is more tied into her brain than her genitalia. If she lacks strong urges for sexual contact, a woman must be more intentional in fostering an awareness of her sexuality. It's the essence of being the subject of your sex life – taking more responsibility and actively nurturing your sexual self.

Becoming the subject of your sex life means:

- Becoming a sexual being with your own sexual needs, feelings, and desires
- Learning to express your sexual needs, feelings, and desires
- Making peace with your body and learning to be *in* your body
- Taking responsibility for nurturing your sexual desire
- Setting, voicing, and enforcing clear sexual boundaries
- Learning to manage differences in sexual desire in a relationship

- Developing a language and comfort in discussing sexual issues
- Respecting the sexual boundaries of others

If the primary experience of your sexuality has been as a sexual object, then you've never fully experienced yourself as a sexual being. You may have been very sexual – responsive to your partner's touch, adventurous in your lovemaking, easily orgasmic, maybe even promiscuous – but still be disconnected from your sexual self. Your sexual feelings and sexual satisfaction may have taken a back seat to the more primary objectives of securing male attention and affection. Your sexual behavior has often focused more on meeting your partner's needs than on exploring and fulfilling your own.

> During Dana's promiscuous phase, she was probably viewed by some as a "nymphomaniac" or a "sex fiend". She certainly engaged in a lot of sexual behavior and faked pleasure she didn't feel. The truth, as Dana tells it, is that most of those liaisons were far from satisfying – at least in the sex department. She enjoyed the touching, kissing, and being held, and she enjoyed feeling wanted and desired. She also enjoyed pleasing her partner and focusing on his satisfaction, but she was rarely orgasmic, herself. The encounters lacked a sense of safety and security, which inhibited relaxation. But Dana's focus for herself was more on securing attention and affection and less on sexual satisfaction, anyway.

Of course, like many women, Dana faked complete satisfaction during even the most casual sexual encounters. As a sexual object, pleasing the one you're with is an important part of the job – and that includes making them believe they've pleased you.

## Orgasm – or Not?

Do men ever wonder why so many women fake orgasm – even women who are normally orgasmic? It's certainly not a widespread phenomenon in the male world. Women who 'fake it' may be taking care of themselves if they're anxious for a sexual encounter to be over, but more often than not, it's about protecting their partner's ego when an orgasm just doesn't feel possible or likely. In order for most women to climax, they first have to relax and tune out distractions. Only then can they focus on the pleasurable physical sensations that increase arousal – and that's easier said than done. Even female rats have difficulty with focus during sex. In the book, *The Sexual Behavior in the Human Female,* Alfred Kinsey reports: "Cheese crumbs spread in front of a copulating pair of rats may distract the female, but not the male." That's why children who are not yet asleep or overnight guests in the house can easily break concentration and disrupt a female's arousal. Anxious thoughts are another disruption. When a woman is worried about how to get her mom to take her meds correctly or whether to respond to a snippy email from her boss, sexual responsiveness can completely shut down. Faking an orgasm avoids the possibility of a partner personalizing the lack of response.

Even without distractions, orgasm can be a problem. About 10% of women have never been orgasmic during sex with their partner, and as many as 25% are rarely orgasmic. Many women who are unable to have an orgasm during intercourse, however, can easily reach orgasm with manual or oral stimulation. Female sexual response is varied and complex, and difficulties with arousal and orgasm can be both a cause and effect of low sexual desire.

Arousal and orgasm are extremely unlikely if there is any pain during sex. Painful intercourse is not uncommon for women on an occasional basis, and about 15% of women experience it on a chronic basis. Pain can be caused by infection, inadequate lubrication, and prolonged, vigorous thrusting during intercourse. A gynecological evaluation is the first step in the treatment of the problem. Lubricants such as Slippery Stuff and Astroglide can be helpful in eliminating discomfort for women with inadequate lubrication, which is an increasing problem as women age. When a woman begins to feel pain or irritation during intercourse, she needs to communicate with her partner. An unknowing partner may be extending his thrusts to bring her to orgasm and can be unaware that he's pushing her further and further away from arousal.

Women who are reluctant to ask for what they want and need and who worry about 'taking too long' may also be inclined to fake orgasm. Many females are not well-versed in their own sexual responsiveness and may not know that the average woman needs 20-30 minutes of stimulation in order to reach orgasm. Apparently a lot of men aren't aware of that need, either. Surveys indicate that a typical sexual encounter involves 15 minutes of foreplay and an additional 5 minutes from the time of penetration to the man's orgasm. It's not surprising, then, that the top three sexual complaints from women are lack of foreplay, unimaginative sex, and a partner reaching orgasm too quickly. Although women may voice these complaints, many still feel they're putting too much of a burden on their partner if the need for foreplay becomes too extended. In addition, reaching orgasm may not be as important to her as it is to her partner.

When an orgasm is the holy grail of every sexual encounter, it creates pressure that works against the body's natural sexual responses. Trying to *make* something happen frequently reduces the probability that it's *going* to happen. Because women are less goal driven in the sexual arena, it's possible for many sexual as well as non-sexual needs to be met in an encounter without ever achieving orgasm. Studies indicate that only one in four women regularly has an orgasm during intercourse. If women were more in touch with their sexuality, that statistic would probably change, but that's not to say that sex without orgasm can't be satisfying. Faking orgasm, on the other hand, can be harmful because it introduces dishonesty into the most intimate of times with your partner, limits your ability to get your needs met, and keeps you in the role of sexual object. It also convinces men that they're much better lovers than they actually are.

When women sacrifice their own satisfaction in sexual encounters by faking it, their partners are free to focus primarily on their own gratification without guilt or remorse. A vicious cycle ensues in which a woman finds little or no pleasure in sex, and her partner – believing her to be satisfied – does nothing that will help change her experience. Both men and women have a role in changing this unhealthy sexual dynamic. For women, it begins with taking more responsibility for their sexual response and becoming more aware of themselves as sexual beings. It is only when a woman is able to clearly specify her erotic preferences, spell out the conditions under which she's comfortable having sex, and claims the right to have her sexual needs met that she will be easily and regularly orgasmic.

**Appeasement and Tradeoff Sex**

In my work as a therapist with both individuals and couples, I frequently hear women say they just don't care about sex, they wouldn't care if they never had sex again, and they have sex with their partners just to appease them because there's a price for on-going avoidance. As one woman told me, "I know when I need to have sex with Larry. The tension just reaches a point where I know if I don't give in, he'll pull away and stop talking to me. He can pout for days."

Appeasement sex is often initiated by women when they notice their partner becoming increasingly tense or cranky from not 'getting any'. Sex is offered as a kind of tranquilizer or mood stabilizer that will relax their partner and put them in a better frame of mind for days afterward. The problem with sex that's dispensed like valium to 'soothe the savage beast' is that it lacks mutuality and intimacy. A sexually hungry partner is probably not going to turn down tranquilizer sex but is unlikely to feel any long-lasting satiation of their hunger because they're hungry for a lot more than sex. As I once heard a man complain, "I swear, I think she's composing a grocery list in her head when we're having sex. I guess I should be happy that she doesn't turn me down, but I'd be just about as happy getting myself off. It feels pretty much the same." There's little joy in lovemaking when women, lacking any interest, merely 'go along' in order to accommodate a partner's physical need. That doesn't mean a woman has to be equally interested at the outset or even equally invested in reaching peak sexual enjoyment at any point in the encounter for sex to be good. It simply means that joyful sex requires engagement and the ability to be fully present. Without that engagement, sex can be a lonely and isolating experience.

Tradeoff sex has similar drawbacks. I once heard a woman say that if she wanted her husband to paint a room, she'd initiate a sizzling sexual encounter the night before and then hit him with her request the next morning. Maybe he never made the connection – or maybe he did, but thought it was a good trade. In either case, when sex is used as a negotiation or a bargaining tool, the loving and open context of giving and receiving is destroyed. Hidden agendas and tradeoffs not only sabotage a couple's sex life, they also compromise the intimacy of the entire relationship

## Medical Issues

There's a wide range of sexual desire in both men and women. Women with low sexual desire may be so for any number of reasons – inhibition, depression, history of sexual abuse, discomfort with their bodies, fatigue, low levels of free testosterone, anger, and relationship problems. Over the last 40 years, women's sexuality has taken an additional hit from the widespread use of birth control pills, as well as from the tremendous increase in the number of hysterectomies performed in the U.S. Medications for the treatment of depression, high blood pressure, and high cholesterol have also become more widely prescribed, all of which have some potential to affect sexual desire and sexual responsiveness.

## Antidepressants

Popular antidepressants, especially the SSRIs (selective serotonin reuptake inhibitors), have done more than dampen the negative effects of depression – they've dampened sexual appetites, as well. Depression, itself, typically wreaks havoc on libido, and it seems a cruel irony that the treatment for depression can cause not only a loss of interest in sex but also difficulty in achieving sexual satisfaction. Not everyone taking antidepressant medication experiences sexual problems. However, if you're experiencing sexual side effects from your antidepressant, you should talk to your doctor about solutions. The doctor may prescribe another medication with a lower risk of sexual dysfunction.

**Other Medications**

Drugs that treat high blood pressure and high cholesterol also carry the potential for interfering with sexual desire. In addition, certain antihistamine medications, diuretics, painkillers, and prescription acid blockers may impact sexual functioning. If you think that any medication you're taking is impairing your sexuality, it's important to talk to your medical provider.

**The Pill**

The very thing that helped spark the sexual revolution has ironically contributed to declining sexual interest. Birth control pills are used by almost 12 million women in the United States, and about 1 in 4 of those women will experience some negative sexual side effect. The negative effects include decreased sexual desire, greater difficulty with arousal, and decreased lubrication. It seems there are two ways that birth control pills may interfere with sexual functioning. The pills block testosterone production in the ovaries and stimulate the production of a protein that decreases the amount of free testosterone in the blood. Even more disturbing, a new study suggests that the sexual side effects of the pill may continue for months after a woman stops taking it. There is even a question about whether the changes induced by the pill are ever completely reversible after discontinued use. There has been very little research done on how hormonal methods of birth control impact a woman's sexuality. For now, women who are suffering from sexual dysfunction related to pill use may want to consider alternative methods of birth control.

## Hysterectomies

A friend of mine whose ovaries were removed a few years ago described the impact on her sex drive:

> "I used to feel like a really sexual person. My husband and I usually had sex two or three times a week, and I initiated it as often as he did. After my surgery, I still enjoyed sex, but my drive just bottomed out. I never think about sex anymore, and I really have to push myself to get in the mood. I feel bad that my husband is always the one that has to get things going. My drive is just gone."

Hysterectomy is the second most frequently performed major surgical procedure for women of reproductive age in the United States, second only to cesarean section. By the age of 60, one out of every three women in the U.S. has had a hysterectomy, which greatly exceeds the rate at which the procedure is performed elsewhere in the world. It seems that American doctors have utilized hysterectomies as a quick and easy fix for 'female problems'.

Of greater concern here is that among women who had a hysterectomy between the years of 1994 and 1999, 55% also had their ovaries removed. In 40% of the cases, the women were less than 45 years old at the time of the procedure. Since 1965, the percentage of women whose hysterectomies also included the removal of the ovaries has doubled.

Why are those statistics significant in understanding low desire? Because the removal of the ovaries is the equivalent of male castration! Removal of both ovaries causes an immediate 50% reduction in circulating testosterone, and a more than 80% drop in circulating estrogen. Both testosterone and estrogen play a vital role in both sexual desire and sexual functioning. When left in place, the ovaries produce hormones long after menopause and support healthy sexual response and performance.

Testosterone directly affects the brain and increases libido. Testosterone also affects mood. Women whose hormones are being produced by their own ovaries have a lower rate of depression than women who have had their ovaries removed, even if hormone replacement therapy (HRT) is taken. Hormone production is a complex process, and it's not surprising that HRT often falls short in replicating and maintaining normal hormone levels. Many women whose ovaries have been removed aren't even taking hormones because of the controversy over HRT and the possible link to breast and ovarian cancer. Those who are will still experience a decline in circulating testosterone. Hormone balance is fragile and complex, and hormonal changes can have a significant impact on sexuality.

If you struggle from low desire as a result of low testosterone, there are options for boosting testosterone levels. Talk to your doctor to see if you're a good candidate for a testosterone gel that is available by prescription. Hopefully, as women's sexual desire begins to be taken more seriously, there will be more options for treating testosterone deficiency. But medical intervention is only a small part of the story. Women can begin now to explore the many non-medical strategies for boosting their desire. The exploration begins with discovering the motivation.

## Sex – Relationship Velcro

In a recent survey, 53% of American women said they preferred shopping to sex. For women who are asking, "Why is sex such a big deal?", "what if I don't want to be a more sexual person?", or "how can I make myself feel something that I don't feel?", the motivation to address the lack of desire may be found in the yearning for more intimacy in a relationship.

If you're in a relationship with someone who cares about sex, that's reason enough for *you* to care about sex. I'm not talking here about 'submitting' to sex or gritting your teeth until the dirty deed is done. What I *am* talking about is taking your partner's needs seriously rather than just 'going along with it'. If you value your partner's needs and wants as much as you value your own, you just can't dismiss, trivialize, or ignore something as important as his sexual desire – even when your own is lacking.

Sex is part of the attachment mechanism that holds your relationship together. It's the one thing that distinguishes a romantic relationship from all others. Oxytocin, the chemical that's released when you're having sex (and when you're breast feeding) is the bonding chemical. Just as it does for a mother and her new baby, oxytocin builds trust and increases connection when released during intimate contact. Let sex slip away from your relationship, and emotional distance usually begins to creep in. Sex is part of the intimacy exclusively shared by a couple. There is real vulnerability in being naked, skin to skin, with another human being and even more vulnerability at the point of orgasm. It's in our willingness to be open and exposed with our partner that we give intimacy a chance to flourish.

So, if I've convinced you to tune into your sexuality, how do you find the station? In Chapter 10, I'll cover some techniques for keeping your sexual energy in high gear. The primary goal here is to first focus on strategies that will help you discover, explore and claim your sexuality.

## Sensuality

Sensuality pertains to gratification through the senses and is a good inroad to your sexuality. Start with what you already do that's sensual, and exaggerate those aspects of your everyday life. For example, pay close attention to the sensations of walking barefoot through the grass, eating a perfectly ripe peach, smelling a moonflower at dusk, petting your cat, relaxing in a hot bath, climbing in between freshly laundered sheets, nursing your baby, slow-dancing with your partner, savoring every bite of that chocolate raspberry cheesecake, taking a walk in a softly falling snow, or coming in from the cold to a cup of hot tea and a crackling fire. If you're not having many sensual experiences, then begin looking at how to increase the delights for your senses. It might help to imagine what you would miss if you lost the ability to see, hear, taste, smell, or feel. I have a sister-in-law who has lost her ability to smell, and the sadness of her experience has increased my appreciation for the smells of cookies baking in the oven, the fragrance from the roses in my garden, and the scent of a freshly cut lime.

A sensuality journal is a good tool to help you begin connecting to your senses. Every night, record at least five positive sensory experiences you've noticed during the day. As your awareness increases, you'll not only develop a new appreciation for the life-enhancing capacity of sensory stimulation, but you may also find yourself seeking more sensory pleasure.

In order to expand your awareness of the sensual experiences in your life, you not only need to tune into your five senses, you also need to slow down. When your mind is constantly bombarded with a frantic rehearsal of the next 24 hours, you miss out on the richness of the moment. Even washing the dishes can be a sensual experience if you're tuned into your senses and remain present in the moment rather than rushing through the chore to get the kids' bedtime routine started. The art of focused awareness is mindfulness – it reduces stress, keeps you present-centered, and helps you maximize the joy in your experiences. In learning how to tune out distractions and be more mindful, you'll also improve your ability to pay close attention to physical sensations. In a study reported by Mary Roach in *Bonk*, women with arousal difficulties noticed a significant increase in how aroused they felt during sexual encounters after they participated in mindfulness training.

How does sensuality then become an inroad to sexuality? By being tuned into your senses and staying more present in the moment, you increase your presence in your body, and you learn the many delights the body has to offer. You also refine your searching image for sex and enhance your capacity for engagement in the physical pleasures sex has to offer.

**Tuning into the Body**

Women are notorious for ignoring very basic physical needs as long as they possibly can. How often do you feel the urge to urinate but delay acting on that urge for anywhere from a few minutes to a few hours? How often do you ignore your hunger and skip meals? How often do you keep working long past the point of mental and physical exhaustion? Men sometimes ignore body signals, too, but women are generally much guiltier of neglecting their bodies. Men are pretty good at getting most of their physical needs met (sex often being one of the exceptions), in part because they were not conditioned to be as self-sacrificing as women. Women delay meeting their physical needs because they often perceive other things – or other people's needs – as more important than their own. But what could be more important than meeting the most basic needs of the body?

We took an informal poll of male and female therapists at an agency where I once worked and asked them if they would excuse themselves from a therapy session if they felt the need to urinate. None of the male therapists even hesitated before saying that they would interrupt a session to heed nature's call. All of the female therapists, however, said they would "hold it" until the end of the session.

Women have been crippled by the tendency to make their needs a low priority. If women have learned to routinely ignore the body's signals for primary physical needs, what is the likelihood that they will be tuned in and responsive to the often subtle signals of sexual interest? Female arousal is complex and involves an intricate set of connections between mind and body. Mary Roach discovered some interesting research which measured the arousal responses of both sexually functional and dysfunctional groups of women to erotic film clips. The women who were dysfunctional differed not in the physical changes that took place in their bodies while watching the clips, but in their *awareness* of the changes. The functional women were more able to notice and pay attention to their responses. Because it's *perceived* arousal that feeds sexual interest, it's important for women to be clued into what's going on in their bodies. However, women's general disregard for their physical selves is further compromised by their difficulty with body acceptance.

## Body Discomfort

Women are prone to dissociating from their bodies because of their incredible body-hatred. If you despise your cellulite-ridden thighs, your pot belly, and your sagging breasts, the easiest thing to do is split off body awareness so that you don't have to feel the shame and inadequacy of your imperfect figure. But that dissociation is often one more reason many women are out of touch with their sexuality.

In addition to disconnecting women from their physical selves, poor body image also has a direct impact on whether women are comfortable engaging in sex. Body discomfort can make sex a downright distasteful experience. Women look in the mirror and zero in with disgust on their hated body parts. They imagine their partner seeing them naked and feeling that same level of repulsion even though men, in general, seem to be much less critical of imperfect bodies. Men tend to appraise their own bodies less critically than women appraise theirs – which is why the guy with the huge beer belly can appear in public in a speedo – and men have been shown to rate their partners as more attractive than those same women rate themselves. But even if a woman knows her partner finds her attractive, she still has to find a way to make peace with her imperfections and find value in her flawed body in order to become a full sexual being. A friend of mine, tired of feeling shame about her body, wrote a poem expressing what she wished a partner would say to her. She decided to say it to herself:

To Myself

I have loved your mind; your restlessly seeking intellect,
And I have loved your spirit, your often down, never
defeated, pragmatic, idealistic, loving, laughing soul.
But in this moment, I love your body.

I love the silky soft touch of your skin;
the ever changing hues of your hazel brown eyes...
I love your generous hips and voluptuous thighs,
and oh, how I celebrate the miracle of their meeting place --
So much more than a vertex -- complete in itself, yet able to
yield and stretch
to hold securely in its upper chamber
a tiny cell, or three kilograms of burgeoning life --
Or, down below, the love and passion of a man.

I worship your shiny dark hair for adorning this sacred
place,
And your rounded tummy, so reminiscent of the lives and
loves you have carried and let go
only to invite another.
I cherish your softly drooping breasts -- no longer resilient,
nor yet nurturing new life;
They still hold comfort and compassion beyond measure.

In this moment, as I trace the lines of worry and thought and joy in your face,
In this moment, I love your body.

Kate Brown '07
(Reprinted with permission of author)

Body hatred leads to inhibited expressions of sexuality, and sexual inhibitions are a much bigger turn-off to a partner than any flab or sagging flesh could ever be. Just remember – it isn't a perfect body that makes you sexy. It's self-confidence and 'moxy'. Men are visual, yes, but their vision doesn't microscopically focus on cellulite or saddle bags. They're focused on *naked* and *hot for me*. The majority of men would kill for the opportunity to ogle the naked body of the woman they love as a prelude to hot, steamy sex.

As a final reflection on body discomfort, my husband and I honeymooned at a Jamaican resort which had a nude beach and a 'clothed' beach. Interestingly enough, the young, hot-bodied guests stuck to their bikinis and speedos on the clothed beach while the nude beach was sparsely populated by the very imperfect bodies of those in their 30's, 40's and beyond - including my husband and me. Those of us who were able to accept ourselves in all our flawed glory and feel comfortable in our skin, were able to fully embrace the delicious joy of swimming and snorkeling naked in the crystal clear waters of the Caribbean.

## Body Acceptance

Body acceptance can be enhanced by regular sessions in front of a full length mirror – naked. Though I know that's a painful experience for many women and one that's avoided by most, it's through exposure that you reach acceptance. Think about your face and how you see it in the mirror every day – often several times in a day. Unless you're one of the fortunate few, you probably recognize facial flaws. Maybe your nose is too big or your eyes are set too far apart or you have a receding chin. Despite the imperfections in your face, you have probably reached a much higher acceptance level of your facial features than you have of your body. You might wish you looked different, but you don't immediately launch an attack on yourself every time you see your face in the mirror. That's where you need to get with your body in order to reach a place of comfort inside your skin.

You can also increase your comfort by shifting your focus from the outside of your body to the inside where your life energy resides. How do you make that shift? Eckhart Tolle in his book, *A New Earth,* suggests closing your eyes and placing your attention on a particular part of the body, such as your hands or feet. Keep your attention there until you can feel the energy, and then move your attention around to different body parts, including your genitals. See if you can feel a tingling or warmth there. Awareness of the inner body is a path to sexual feelings and a sense of your own sexual aliveness.

Another way to increase body awareness and learn to fully inhabit your body is through physical movement. Any kind of physical exercise – walking, running, swimming, lifting weights, gardening, dancing, skating – will help keep you from being a 'walking head' – a brain cut off from everything below the neck. Just being more conscious of the way your body moves you through your daily activities will help you stay connected to your physical being.

Exercise, tone up, change what you can, but begin to appreciate all that your body does for you and stop waging a war with it. Begin relating to yourself more lovingly. See the parts you dislike through a lens of compassion rather than a lens of judgment. Feel your energy and breath move freely throughout your body. Feel the space that you occupy and stretch out to fully fill up that space. Start heeding the physical signals that you're receiving: urinate when you first feel the urge; eat when you're hungry; sleep when you're tired. And, very importantly, notice even the smallest flickering of sexual desire.

### Genital Self Image and Acceptance

Has it come to your attention that the average man seems to have a love affair going on with his penis? He plays with it, whips it out at the slightest invitation (and sometimes without an invitation), shakes it at his partner when toweling off after a shower, and walks around naked with a sense of pride. Wouldn't it be wonderful if women had the same kind of love for their vulvas? According to sex therapist, Dr. Laura Berman, positive thoughts about our genitals are essential to self-acceptance and sexual growth. At the Berman Center, she found that women with more positive genital self-images were found to have more sexual desire and better sexual response. This means they reported more lubrication during sexual activity and better quality orgasms. In fact, they were six times more likely to have a good sex life than women with poor genital self-image.

Unlike men, women's genitals are a more covert operation. Not only are they more hidden, females are discouraged from exploring their genitalia. With little reference point for comparison, women may wonder if their genitals are 'normal'. So how do women begin claiming, celebrating, and connecting to their genitals? First, they need to know what they look like. The advice of early feminists to look at your genitals with a hand mirror is still sound. Women's genitals come in lots of shapes and sizes, and symmetry is not always the rule. Variation in the layout of the outer and inner labia, as well as in the appearance of the clitoris, is normal. Women need to accept their genitals as they are if they're going to have a healthy sexual identity.

The discomfort many women feel with their genitals may have less to do with appearance and more to do with fears or concerns about discharge. All women have vaginal discharge because the vagina produces secretions to cleanse itself and to provide lubrication that makes sex comfortable and enjoyable. The scent connected with the vagina is natural and may actually be a turn-on for a woman's partner. Offensive odors are often caused by yeast and bacterial infections, which usually require medical attention. The risk of infection can be minimized by keeping the vulva clean and dry. Thorough drying after washing discourages the growth of bacteria, as does wearing cotton panties.

It's pretty tough to feel good about your sexuality unless you feel good about your genitals. Becoming more familiar with your sexual anatomy and appreciating its complexity will help you embrace and celebrate this important part of your body.

## Sexual Learning

First learning to accept and fully inhabit your body will help you tune into your body's sexual responses. Next, if you haven't already done it, it's important to learn about your erogenous zones. Though there are certain parts of the body that are more loaded with nerve endings than others and are very responsive to touch for the majority of people, each person is unique in terms of erotic preferences. What is a real turn-on for one person might drive another person crazy. The list of possible erogenous zone is extensive – ears, neck, scalp, lips, nipples, breasts, thighs, clitoris, vulva, vagina, buttocks, anus, feet, toes, hands, fingers – and each area may be capable of arousing different sexual feelings. Identifying the areas of your body that are most sexually responsive is an important step out of passivity and will give you more control over activating your desire.

Information is vital in giving up the role of sexual object. Sensate focus exercises are those in which you and your partner take turns giving and receiving touch all over your bodies without the goal of intercourse or orgasm. Sensitive touching accompanied by feedback can help you and your partner figure out what feels good and what doesn't. Once you identify your particular erogenous zones, the next step is to identify what kind of touch is desired in those areas. Do you like kissing, licking, stroking – light pressure, firm pressure – repetitive or intermittent? And when do you desire touch – early on in the sexual encounter, in the middle, or only when fully stimulated? What is the quickest way for you to get turned on? How do you most easily reach orgasm? Are there certain sexual positions which make it easier for you to reach orgasm? Some of these questions will only be answered in conjunction with your partner, but by stimulating your own erogenous zones and by masturbating, you can discover a lot about the kind of touch that brings you sexual pleasure and satisfaction. It's also helpful to pay attention to the images and fantasies that enhance your self-pleasuring. They may contain important information about the kind of sexual interactions that intensify your sexual enjoyment. Learning to maximize your pleasure will help create the kind of sex you'll want to return to on a regular basis.

Another inroad to your sexuality can be found in Kegels, an exercise designed to strengthen the muscles that form part of the pelvic floor. These are the same muscles used to stop the flow of urine, and can be easily identified in that way. Flexing your pelvic floor muscles mimics the contractions of orgasm and can increase genital sensitivity and blood flow to the pelvis, as well as produce stronger orgasms. For women, Kegels are one of the quickest ways to access sexual feelings. By doing them regularly, you can stay in touch with your sexuality on a daily basis. You can also do a few Kegels to help prepare you for sexual activity when your interest level is low. So, do the squeezes to tone up and increase sexual pleasure for both you and your partner, but also keep them in mind the next time you need a quick desire-starter.

Part of claiming your sexuality is taking responsibility for your own desire. A passage from *Black Water*, a novel by Joyce Carol Oates, illustrates how passively some women experience their desire:

> "As he kissed her those several times, kissing, sucking, groping…she felt the jolt of desire: not her desire, but the man's. As, since girlhood, kissing and being kissed, Kelly Kelleher had always felt, not her own, but the other's, the male's, desire. Quick and galvanizing as an electric shock. Feeling too, once she caught her breath, that familiar wave of anxiety, guilt – I've made you want me, now I can't refuse you."

Until women can learn to focus on and activate their own desire, they won't be fully in charge of their sexuality.

## Z-z-z-z-z-z-z-z-z

The final recommendation in the physical realm has to do with sleep. A good number of Americans, both male and female, operate with too little sleep, but women are especially prone to shaving off hours of sleep either at night or in the morning in order to get everything done. Many of my female clients are still up when the rest of the household has gone to bed, doing one last load of laundry or finishing a report for work, and I know many women who are up by 5:00 a.m. to squeeze in a little exercise before entering the rush of the daily routine. These are often the same women who tell me, "When I hit the bed at night, the last thing on my mind is fooling around under the covers. All I want to do is sleep – and I don't want him to even think about trying something in the middle of the night!" If you are always tired, you can't expect to have much interest in sex, so it's imperative to find a way to get more sleep. Even if it means putting off the laundry for another day and going without underwear – sleep must become a high priority. It's also crucial to get in charge of your stress because no amount of sleep is going to revive you if you're stressed to the max every day. Stress will not only zap your sex drive as quickly as fatigue, it's a major source of fatigue.

## Claiming Power

Getting your physical life in order is both rejuvenating and empowering. So once you've claimed more physical power for yourself, it's time to claim power in your relationship. I'm always amazed by the number of strong, assertive women who give up their power in a primary relationship. These women run companies and perform heart surgery and organize major community events, yet they easily relinquish their voice with their partner. If you don't express your wants and needs outside the bedroom, you'll certainly be very unlikely to express them inside the bedroom. And if you're not asking for what you want and need, whether that's a back rub or more help with the housework, you're probably building resentment – the sure-fire desire killer.

Claiming power not only helps you get your needs met, it's also critical to intimacy. Real intimacy – both emotional and physical – only takes place between equals. Maintaining a balance of power in the relationship is, therefore, essential if intimacy is going to thrive. If it's conflict avoidance or your partner's anger that keeps you from claiming power, it's important for you to begin facing those fears. You may need the help of a therapist if you feel paralyzed and unable to take the first steps. Couple's therapy can be useful in helping you and your partner find safe and constructive ways of managing conflict. Don't wait until your relationship is on life-support before seeking help. You have more to lose than your sex life.

Jean A. Campbell

## Final Thoughts

Women face many challenges on their journey from sex object to sex subject. It begins by questioning the programming that emphasizes passivity, self-sacrifice, and desirability rather than desire. It continues with the difficult task of accepting and tuning into a body that doesn't measure up to Madison Avenue's idealized female figure. Then there's also overcoming inhibition to learn how that body responds to specific sexual stimulation. Finally, it's stepping up to the plate and claiming power – power within a relationship and power to determine the real meaning of 'sexy'. The process of taking sexy back begins when women are in touch with both the lioness as well as the lamb contained in their femininity.

# Exercise

Are you the subject of your sex life? Rate yourself on the following items and see where you might still need some work. 1 is 'not true' and 5 is 'very true'.

1. I'm comfortable with my body and stay tuned into it    1   2   3   4   5

2. I have spontaneous feelings of sexual desire    1   2   3   4   5

3. I share my sexual wants and needs with my partner    1   2   3   4   5

4. I feel sexy    1   2   3   4   5

5. I create feelings of desire by reading sexy books and fantasizing    1   2   3   4   5

6. I know how I can most easily reach orgasm    1   2   3   4   5

7. I sometimes initiate sex with my partner    1   2   3   4   5

8. I'm comfortable in turning down sex with my partner    1   2   3   4   5

9. I'm comfortable discussing sex with my partner    1   2   3   4   5

10. I never fake orgasms    1   2   3   4   5

11. I value the sexual part of my relationship    1   2   3   4   5

12. I get regular physical exercise    1   2   3   4   5

13. I do a good job of meeting my body's physical needs    1   2   3   4   5

14. I know exactly where and how I like to be touched    1   2   3   4   5

15. I'm comfortable sharing fantasies with my partner    1   2   3   4   5

16. I sometimes masturbate    1   2   3   4   5

17. I do Kegels on a regular basis    1   2   3   4   5

18. I express my wants and needs in my relationship   1   2   3   4   5

19. I have equal decision-making power in my relationship   1   2   3   4   5

20. I often try new things and strive to be happy   1   2   3   4   5

# Chapter 5

## Mission Possible:
## When One Head Isn't Working, Use the Other

A husband and wife were retiring for the night. Soon after they both climbed into bed, the husband got up, went to the bathroom, and got a glass of water and two aspirin. He took the water and aspirin over to his wife's side of the bed and said, "Here you go, honey." The wife looked at him quizzically and replied, "But I don't have a headache." The husband smiled and said, "That's just what I wanted to hear."

Most jokes about marital sex have a similar theme – the sex-starved husband who begs, pleads, and pressures his disinterested wife to get a little action in the sack. The stereotype of the 'always ready to go' man is still hanging around. But these days, I'm just as likely to hear the following story:

"Early on in our marriage, my wife and I had a great sex life. We both liked to try new things, and we never seemed to get bored with each other. Then we went through a bad spell with our teenage son who'd gotten heavily involved in drugs, and it seemed like all of our energy and attention was focused on dealing with him. I was also feeling a lot more pressure with my job during those years, and my wife and I just gradually grew apart. Worse than that, we began taking our stress out on each other, and eventually it seemed like all we ever did was argue or give each other the silent treatment. We haven't had sex in almost a year, and truthfully, I don't even miss it anymore. I don't really have the energy or the interest – and at this point, I don't know how we'd get past the awkwardness to get back to where we used to be with each other."

Many men, as well as women, are floundering in the desire department. We just don't often hear from these men because they're embarrassed to admit they might prefer a night in front of the TV to a roll in the hay. A man's masculinity is very tied into his sexual feelings and sexual functioning. When a boy hits adolescence, the presence of desire is hard to miss, and the erections that pop up at the slightest provocation (and often even without any provocation) are a sure sign that the boy is becoming a man. The sex drive is so powerful during adolescence that it is defining.

Females don't have this external, commanding body part signaling sexual desire and don't generally equate their femininity with feelings of desire. In fact, as discussed in the last chapter, a woman's femininity is much more tied into whether or not she feels *desired* rather than desiring. Her desire never assumes center stage, so if later in life it's minimal or missing in action, it isn't as shameful for her to admit. When desire wanes, she doesn't feel less like a woman. She may, however, suffer a serious blow to her self esteem when she no longer feels *desirable*.

In fact, I often hear about low desire men initially from their partners who come in complaining of feeling disconnected and disengaged in their relationships. Even low desire women complain about the absence of passion in their relationships and describe their partners disparagingly as "roommates". They no longer feel attractive or desirable to their mates. They miss the touching and affection even if they don't miss the sex, and they mourn the loss of closeness that sex once provided. Their partners have stopped initiating sex and find excuses to avoid it if the opportunity arises. In a typical scenario, the partner comes home tired from work and sits in front of the television or computer screen for hours after dinner. He may have several beers and fall asleep on the couch by 9:00 p.m. His partner describes him as a "slug", and, if he's lost his passion, it may be a pretty accurate description. Sue is married to one of these men:

> "He doesn't want to do anything anymore. Even when I suggest going out to dinner, he just wants me to go out and bring something back. He doesn't look at me or notice if I'm wearing something new. He didn't even say a word when I came home from the hairdresser with 6 inches chopped off my hair. I have

to admit, it got me thinking about a different 6 inches I could chop off! I'm sure that would get his attention – though he hasn't been using those 6 inches on me. I feel invisible. Now I understand why people have affairs – compared to the blob I have sitting at home, just about every guy I run into looks good."

## What Happened?

How did this guy who was once a walking hard-on become so apathetic about sex? Even though men have 10 to 100 times more testosterone than women, they are still subject to many of the same desire-killers. Antidepressants, stress, fatigue, medications for high blood pressure and diabetes, depression, low self esteem, and leading a mind-numbing existence can all take a significant toll on a man's sex drive. Most men are also subject to at least occasional problems with getting or sustaining an erection, and it's estimated that over 25 million men suffer from impotence on a regular basis. Men often delay seeking treatment because of embarrassment or a belief that the problem will eventually just go away. However, during that delay, a destructive pattern of sexual avoidance and decreased desire often sets in. Since men are typically expected to take the lead in initiating sexual activity and are under more pressure to perform when it occurs, it's important to take a closer look at how some of these factors specifically affect men and their relationships.

## Medications

Medications, including antidepressants, can have a deadening effect on sexual desire and may also make it more difficult for a man to reach orgasm. Though both men and women on medication may struggle with these side effects, the impact on men's sexuality is often more profound. The greater impact is due in part to the blow a man takes to his masculinity when he loses desire. Intercourse is also more dependent upon his performance than on his partner's. With the right lubrication, a woman can have intercourse whether she's feeling much desire or not. Men, on the other hand, are dependent upon an erection to have sex. If a man isn't feeling much desire, he may worry about being able to get and maintain an erection. His masculinity may feel compromised if he has to ask his partner for extra stimulation. Even if the erection isn't a problem, orgasm might be. Men are typically more goal focused when it comes to sex, and though both sexes may be equally interested in reaching orgasm, men feel a greater sense of inadequacy when it fails to happen. Intercourse that goes on and on without climax soon becomes frustrating and even painful – for both participants.

Problems with erection and/or orgasm can create embarrassment and shame. The anticipation of experiencing those difficulties often exacerbates the problem and can lead to the avoidance of future sexual encounters. Once a man can no longer rely on his performance being predictable and satisfactory, he may find it easier to stay up late than to risk "failing" again. Unfortunately, the cause of the avoidance is seldom discussed with his partner, and is rarely discussed with a doctor.

This silence compounds the problem. It's important for a man to consult a urologist if he's concerned about the physical dimension of his sexual functioning, as erectile dysfunction can be the first sign of high blood pressure or a blockage in the arteries. The doctor needs to know about the sexual side effects of any medications being prescribed. There may be alternative medications available that have less impact on sexual functioning, or medications may be prescribed to help counteract the impact.

It's also critical for men to talk to their partners about any changes in their level of sexual desire or sexual functioning. If there is difficulty with either erection and/or orgasm, it's important to talk about what your partner might do to help, or what the two of you together might do differently to address the issue. Avoiding sexual contact with a partner when changes occur is a losing proposition for both parties.

Bob started having difficulty with erections after his doctor put him on high blood pressure medication. Luckily, he was able to talk to his partner about his concerns:

> "This is tough for me to talk about, but I don't want our sex life to go to hell just because I can't always count on a solid hard-on. It would help me a lot if you would

use more pressure when you're touching my penis. I also want to satisfy you even when I can't actually have intercourse. Please don't take it personally if I don't come – that just puts more pressure on me which makes the whole problem worse. There are a lot of things we can do in bed even if I can't get hard."

## Erection Anxiety

Normal changes that accompany aging can also create 'failures' that inhibit sexual behavior. Though over 40% of men remain sexually active past the age of 70, over half of healthy males in the 40-70 age range experience some degree of impotence. Episodes of impotence are more likely as a man ages due to a diminished supply of testosterone. But unless there are other factors involved, it's often the man's *response* to the failed erection that creates ongoing difficulty. After experiencing an erectile dysfunction, he begins to have anticipatory anxiety about his performance which tends to produce the failed erections he fears. That, in turn, can lead to increased sexual avoidance.

Further compounding the problem within the relationship is the gradual disappearance of affectionate touch toward his partner. Fearing that his partner may misinterpret kisses and warm embraces as an interest in sex, he begins avoiding physical contact. So now his partner not only isn't getting any sex, but she's also not getting touched. It's small wonder that she begins to feel unwanted and unloved. As one partner avoids and the other feels rejected, both begin shutting down and distancing from one another – a cycle that wreaks havoc in relationships and heaps more stress onto an already stressful situation. Mary, a 53-year-old client, finally realized that she and her husband were caught in that cycle:

> "Of course I noticed that Jack's hard-ons had become less reliable, but it didn't really bother me. What did bother me was the shut-down in physical affection. Jack had always been very affectionate – holding hands, kissing me on the back of the neck when I was washing dishes, snuggling with me on the couch, going to sleep spooning – but ever since we started having trouble in the sex department, he has really pulled back. Once I caught onto the problem, I told Jack that I wanted the affection back. I told him I would leave it up to him if he wanted to go any further, but I was not going to become just roommates."

If you're experiencing sexual difficulties or reduced libido that isn't related to medication side effects or disease, your doctor can perform a test that measures free testosterone levels in your blood. Testosterone replacement therapy is available in pills, injections, a patch, or pellets placed under the skin – all of which are effective in treating testosterone deficiency and can make a big difference in your libido and general sense of well being. Testosterone therapy is not usually effective in treating erection difficulties, but there are several drugs now on the market for the treatment of erectile dysfunction, such as Viagra and Cialis.

The non-medical treatment for erectile dysfunction emphasizes intimacy over erections. Couples can explore non-intercourse focused touch and mutual genital pleasuring. It's helpful if the couple develops realistic expectations and is able to take a waxing and waning erection in stride. Experimentation with different sexual techniques, including more oral and manual stimulation of the penis, is usually beneficial. It's important to take the pressure off the penis, which is not, after all, a perfectly functioning machine. Sex is not performance art – it's about sharing closeness, pleasure, and intimacy. Without preconceived notions about what has to happen in every sexual encounter, a couple can slow down and enjoy the journey rather than focusing on the final destination. Men need to recognize the value in staying physically close and allow intimacy to replace performance as the primary goal of sexual encounters. A relaxed attitude and a sense of humor are also invaluable in keeping a failed erection from becoming a personal or couple failure.

**Chronic Erectile Dysfunction**

Men with chronic, rather than episodic, erectile dysfunction frequently worry about their inability to sexually satisfy their partners, but it's usually a bigger concern for the man than it is for his partner. If you don't trust me on this, trust Ann Landers – remember the question she posed in her column some years ago about sex vs. cuddling? Twenty thousand women wrote in to say that they'd give up intercourse if they could have more hugs and cuddling. The bigger problem for women with an impotent partner tends to be the partner's response to the impotence, which was the case with Bill.

> Bill came in to see me because his doctor had taken him off the Viagra he'd been using to treat his impotence. Humiliated and depressed, Bill couldn't imagine his girlfriend wanting to stay with him if he could no longer perform sexually. He found himself constantly imagining her falling into bed with another man. He no longer felt he had much to offer. His girlfriend *was* starting to get fed up with him, but not because of his sexual problem – she was tired of his jealousy, his hang-dog attitude, and tired of him questioning why she wanted to be with him. Lately, she had begun asking herself that same question.

Bill's challenge was to accept his impotence without it destroying his self esteem. What happened – or didn't happen – during sex wasn't the problem. It was the story that Bill told himself about what it meant to be impotent that was the problem.

**Premature Ejaculation**

Surveys indicate that 3 out of every 10 adult males experience premature ejaculation, which is usually defined as ejaculation that occurs within a minute after intercourse begins or in fewer than 20 strokes. Although this can affect a man's confidence and prove frustrating for his partner, ejaculatory control can be learned. One popular method is a stop-start technique in which the man signals his partner to stop stimulation for 30 to 60 seconds as he nears the point of ejaculation and then signals her to resume stimulation when the urge has passed. The method can be practiced with manual stimulation as well as with intercourse. The female-on-top position is best in facilitating more ejaculatory control.

## Wiped Out

Stress and fatigue are often associated with diminished libido, and they usually go hand in hand. Nothing we do – smoking, drinking, eating too much, not exercising – takes a greater toll on our health than excessive stress. Though some degree of stress is necessary to keep life interesting, excessive stress – *dis*tress – is the norm in our fast-paced culture. We talk about being "stressed out" and "overwhelmed", but we don't stop to take a break and let our bodies recover. We keep on truckin', even though stress is making us tired, irritable, depressed, and sick. Who cares about sex when your tank is near empty?

Actually, before becoming totally depleted, men may try to fill their tank up with sex. I recently heard a woman react quite heatedly when her boyfriend described sex as a "tension release" for him. She felt used. She failed to understand that sex meets multiple needs simultaneously, and that her boyfriend could experience a release of tension, as well as tenderness, caring, and intimacy. The idea of sex as a stress reliever was also quite foreign to her. Women experiencing stress are more likely to *lose* interest in sex rather than gain it. But even men who have an increased sexual interest when under the gun will lose it after being under the gun too long. Then, instead of seeking sex, they begin shutting down, and fatigue and numbness set in. Like a computer in 'sleep' mode, they may be on but not really operational – and depression may soon follow.

Being "stressed out" is not inevitable despite all the balls you're attempting to juggle. Address the sources of stress in your life, and begin making changes today. If it's your job that's eating you alive, find a different way of doing it or find another job. If it's your relationship that's stressing you out, do whatever is necessary to fix it – including couple's therapy, if needed. Your life may depend on it. Carl learned this lesson the hard way – after having a heart attack and undergoing by-pass surgery:

> "I was working 12 hour days and coming home exhausted every night. I knew I wasn't giving much to my marriage, but I still hated my wife's constant harping about how alone she felt. We were only having sex about once a month, if that. Then I had the heart attack and it really shook me up. I realized I wasn't living the life I wanted to live. I found another job – one that I can do in 40-45 hours a week – and I started dating my wife all over again. Now we're having sex at least once a week."

## Depression

Depression destroys your ability to find pleasure in things that were once pleasurable, kills your motivation, disrupts sleep and appetite, and replaces feelings and interest in life with a dull numbness. It basically puts out the fire feeding your passion – your passion for living, as well as your sexual passion. I don't think I've ever talked to a depressed person who reported feeling much, if any, sexual desire. It's usually not even voiced as a major complaint, however, because sex is low on the list of priorities when life feels pointless.

If you're experiencing symptoms of depression, it's important to address the problem. Like many men, you may be reluctant to initiate therapy because you don't like admitting you need help, and you certainly don't like asking for it. Do it anyway. Get started by making an appointment with a therapist recommended by someone you trust. Depression colors every aspect of your life and affects everyone that's close to you. Linda was one of those affected when her husband became depressed. She tried to be supportive, but eventually found herself succumbing to the darkness of Rob's moods.

"When Rob's depression had been going on for a couple of months, I realized that I was sinking into my own black hole. It's like it was contagious, and as hard as I tried to keep my spirits up, I just couldn't do it anymore. If you haven't lived with a depressed person, you have no idea what it's like to endure the silence and apathy and withdrawal. Rob became little more than an empty shell – how could I *not* be depressed?"

Sometimes depression may be a symptom of male menopause or andropause. Though male menopause doesn't affect all men, about 40% of men between 40 and 60 experience many of the same symptoms that women experience during menopause: mood swings, hot flashes, irritability, insomnia, lack of energy, depression, and decreased libido. Male menopause is the result of a slow decline in the production of testosterone after age 40. Fortunately, the decrease is often gradual enough for men to remain sexually active into their 70's, 80's, and beyond. But as they age, it's important for men to stop measuring themselves by their sexual performance and begin focusing on sexual fulfillment. In the second half of life, performance-based sexuality can be a formula for frustration and low self esteem.

### Self Esteem

Low self esteem can also contribute to depression – though it's sometimes hard to figure out which comes first. One certainly feeds the other, and low self esteem also negatively impacts a man's sex drive. There are many forces that erode self esteem as a man ages in addition to the effects of decreasing testosterone. Problems within a relationship are one of the forces that can exact a heavy toll on a man's confidence and sense of self.

It doesn't take anything as dramatic as a partner's affair or a divorce to shred a man's self esteem. Even in a fairly strong relationship, a man can start feeling very down on himself if he's with a low desire partner who frequently rejects his sexual advances. If he's put on some weight, gotten out of shape, or lost most of his hair, he may assume that his partner's disinterest is related to his physical decline. How he responds to feeling rejected may well exacerbate the problem and result in even more distance and coldness in the relationship. It's a negative, frustrating cycle that's disheartening and disempowering.

The inevitable losses that accompany aging and life transitions also carry the potential to lower self esteem. Diminishing physical abilities or chronic pain can bring an increasing sense of vulnerability and weakness that challenge a sense of competence. The loss of a job through layoffs or even a planned and eagerly anticipated retirement can be a hard adjustment as it's often accompanied by greater social isolation and the need to redefine oneself.

Whatever the cause, low self esteem wrecks the confidence that fuels a healthy sexual desire. 'Healthy' is an important qualifier because there *are* men whose low self esteem fuels a sexual neediness. These are men who need sex once or twice a day to reassure them that they are loved and wanted, since they're quite certain they are neither. This is an issue that should be addressed in therapy. But if you're a man whose sex drive has taken a hit as a result of fatigue, erectile dysfunction, stress, or an accumulation of losses, there are strategies for boosting your libido.

## Sexual 'Doing' to Sexual Being

Your programming conditioned you to be a sexual 'doing' – focused primarily on your skill as a lover and the performance of your penis. When your sex drive was intense and your erections reliable, that indoctrination may not have seemed problematic. The problems existed even then, however, and manifested primarily in your intimate relationships. With a strong goal orientation that made orgasm the primary target of sexual encounters, you may have missed the richness of the sexual journey. Even lovers skilled in the mechanics of foreplay have often been more engaged in their own performance than engaged with their partner. Truly making love is less about the right moves and more about *presence*. Presence requires you to be emotionally available to your partner and to be aware of the dynamic exchange of sensual and sexual energy between you. It means bringing all dimensions of your life into the sexual experience rather than just your physical body. When you incorporate your heart and mind into your sexuality, you become a sexual being rather than a sexual 'doing', and you immediately begin to reap the rewards of a fuller and richer sexual life. Greater wholeness as a sexual being not only increases passion and desire, it also changes how you view sexual 'problems'.

## Using Your Head to Boost Your Sex Drive

The brain is our largest and most important sex organ. Fortunately, we have much more control over how we *think* about what happens to us than we have over what actually happens to us. Thoughts drive both feelings and behavior, so by getting in charge of your thoughts, you begin taking charge of your life – and your libido.

> George came into see me at the insistence of his wife who was frustrated by his shut-down at home. He no longer took an interest in projects around the house, had stopped wanting to socialize with friends, was drinking more, and the couple's sex life had dwindled to perfunctory sex once every couple of months. George confessed he was probably depressed. Since turning 50 a few months earlier, he'd begun to focus on his losses and all that he was no longer capable of doing. He'd been forced to drop the tennis he once loved because of bad knees, and he no longer liked what he saw when he looked in the mirror. He'd reached a plateau in his career, and was just putting in his time until retirement. There had also been several times in the last year when he couldn't keep his erection when he and his wife were making love. That last one was a real kicker – the one that made him feel used up and over the hill.

George had fallen into the trap of becoming problem-focused. He'd created a welcome environment for negative thoughts about his life that only helped perpetuate his problems. If he thinks the second half of life sucks, then it does. If he believes he's used up, then he'll shut down and won't bother to figure out how he wants to live for the next 40 years. Until he changes his thoughts, George will not act in a way that will change his circumstances. But how does that work?

To change your thoughts, you start by focusing on your assets rather than on your deficits. Being problem-focused doesn't solve anything – it just keeps you stuck in the problem. Identify what you value about yourself and what you think your partner values about you. Then *ask* your partner what she values about you. You'll probably be surprised to find that it's a lot more than your good looks (or your former good looks). What women find sexy if often very different from what men tend to find sexy since women are less visually focused. This is not to say that women don't admire the Brad Pitts and George Clooneys of the world, but they're just as likely to be attracted to a big, teddy bear kind of man as the guy gracing the cover of GQ. It's self-confidence that's sexy, and being funny, passionate, energetic, and generous.

I can't help but think of Mick Jagger who I recently saw in concert. Mick is skinny, ugly, and old, but raw passion, energy, and intensity make him very sexy – at least in my book. The real turn-on is a man who feels good about himself, who can connect with his partner on multiple levels, who is not overly needy or demanding, and who is engaged in life.

If you're facing the kind of shut-down George experienced,

I'd encourage you to decide that the second half of your life is going to be the best half. I've often thought that the first half of life is like a giant inhalation – we're always sucking up, trying to prove ourselves, and trying to be what other people need us to be. On the other hand, the second half of life is a welcome and gradual exhalation in which we no longer have so much to prove and can finally be who we want to be. There's great freedom and power in knowing who we are, what we want, and why we want it. Priorities are clearer, and there's less angst over the small stuff. We're wiser and maybe even wealthier. More than any other generation before us, we have the chance to redefine mid-life and beyond. Holding onto our passion will both stoke the fires at home and enhance the contributions we make to the world.

## Cranking Up Your Sex Drive

Here are a few more ideas for energizing your sex life:

- Exercise. It's a great antidote for depression, revs up your energy, makes you feel better about yourself, and gets you more in touch with your physical body. Stretching helps maintain flexibility which is important to an active sex life (think yoga or tai chi).
- Watch your drinking. Alcohol is a depressant – and you know what too much alcohol does to your ability to perform sexually. You're also poor company for your partner after you've downed three stiff

drinks and are dozing off in your Lazy Boy. Alcohol interferes with your ability to be engaged and emotionally present.

- Stay excited about something in your life. Whether it's a passion for fly fishing or fixing up old corvettes, a man who's interested and engaged in life is more likely to hold onto his libido – and to activate his partner's libido.

- Identify issues in your relationship that are shutting you down and decide that you're going to do your part to change them. If you feel rejected by your partner and you've shut down in response, then find out what she wants from you. It's amazing how many women warm up to their partners when their needs start getting met – whether that's getting help with the housework, feeling valued outside the bedroom, or having a date night once a week. If you're both waiting for the other to change first, unfortunately, you'll both be waiting forever.

- Just as women can kick start their sexual drive with a hot movie or an erotic novel, men can benefit from this desire-starter, too. We usually think of men's interest in pornography as a *result* of their sex drive, but it certainly doesn't hurt to be intentional about seeking some visual stimulation when the juices aren't flowing on their own. Ideally, you and your partner can watch something together.

**Final Thoughts**

I'm not suggesting that if you follow the guidelines in this chapter, you'll recapture the youthful, carefree vigor of a horny 18-year-old. That's probably a blessing anyway since, unfortunately, you do have to go to work and take out the garbage and answer emails. A man's sexuality changes as he ages. There's less urgency connected to it, which can increase the opportunity for intimacy. Mature sexuality is less about the performance and more about mutual pleasuring. You can have a rich and enjoyable sex life despite the changes and limitations imposed by life circumstances and aging. It's definitely a mission possible.

## *Exercise*

---

If you've been struggling with low desire, consider which of the following may be contributing to your sexual shut-down.

1.  Medications I'm taking which may have sexual side effects:

_____

_____

_____

_____

2.  Erection Anxiety or Premature Ejaculation
    \_\_\_\_\_ I've started avoiding sex because of performance fears
    \_\_\_\_\_ I've pulled back from physical affection with my partner
    \_\_\_\_\_ I haven't talked openly with my partner about my concerns

3.  Wiped Out
    \_\_\_\_\_ I'm overloaded with stress
    \_\_\_\_\_ I'm frequently too tired to even think about sex
    \_\_\_\_\_ I feel numb

4.  Depression
    \_\_\_\_\_ Life often doesn't feel worth living
    \_\_\_\_\_ I don't feel any sexual desire
    \_\_\_\_\_ I'm often irritable and unmotivated

5.  Self Esteem
    \_\_\_\_\_ I don't like what I see in the mirror
    \_\_\_\_\_ I've frequently felt rejected in my relationship
    \_\_\_\_\_ I've experienced losses that make me question my worth

6.  Others

_____

_____

_____

_____

Now take a few minutes to develop a plan for addressing the issues you've identified:

For example,

"I'll make an appointment with my doctor to discuss the sexual side effects of the medication I'm taking."

_____

_____

_____

_____

_____

_____

# Chapter 6

## *Dead in the Water? Desire Killers in Your Midst*

As if bad programming and gender differences aren't enough, lifestyle changes in recent decades have taken their own toll on the sex lives of millions of Americans. The complexities of the modern family, unrealistic expectations of relationships, and the stress associated with a fast-paced, multi-tasking way of life have all waged an assault on desire. We're living in a culture in which the majority of Americans are over-worked and under-sexed. What's happened over the last 50 years to create such a drag on our sex lives?

### Wanting More from Relationships

As if we didn't already have enough to handle, what we began expecting from our primary relationships increased in the last few decades, as well. Many people saw the exploding divorce rate in the 70's as the death knell of marriage. Disillusioned with an institution that promised a lot more than it delivered, more couples than ever began living together without a legal document. But the increase in the number of couples shacking up and the escalation in the divorce rate didn't mean people were giving up on permanent relationships.

They were simply giving themselves an out in case the relationships failed in the 'happily ever after' department. For these members of the "me generation" and the generations that followed, commitment to a partner – 'til death do us part' – had fallen to somewhere below the personal *right* to happiness. And a partner who couldn't make a significant contribution to that happiness by supplying intimacy, fulfillment, and passion might soon find that the permanency of their relationship was more tenuous than they believed. It was no longer enough just to be a good partner who was kind, responsible, and hard-working. Since the 70's, men and women have been increasingly looking for the soul mate who will fill a multitude of needs while maintaining a romantic connection. However, a mounting focus on individualism has actually *de*creased rather than *in*creased the probability of finding such a perfect mate. Couples, lacking the necessary skills to create a healthy relationship and burdened with the personal agendas of both partners, are often experiencing disappointment and despair.

One of my clients who was considering asking her husband for a divorce voiced a laundry list of dissatisfactions and ended the litany with these questions:

> "When is it my turn for happiness? Do I owe him my whole life because of a decision I made when I was too young to know better? Am I just being selfish or do I deserve to have the life that I want? I hate hurting him and I hate what a divorce would do to our kids, but I just don't think I can stay in a marriage that's making me miserable – and I don't think he could ever change enough for me to be happy."

And what about the couples who manage to stick it out? The increased expectations take a toll on them, too. When nudity gives way to flannel pajamas and the demands of children, jobs, household chores, and bills begin battering the relationship, it becomes a lot more difficult to stay connected and happy. As each partner fails to live up to the implicit promises of the courtship, resentment begins to build. Eventually, it finds its way into the bedroom. A vicious cycle soon emerges as decreased sexual contact creates resentment from the higher desire partner, and the lower desire partner responds with distance, anger, and further refusal of sexual overtures. A cold and isolating shutdown often follows. The phrase "I love you, but I'm not *in* love with you anymore" is frequently uttered by at least one of the partners. I've heard some version of the following story far too many times:

> "We just feel like housemates. All we talk about is the kids or who's going to call the plumber. We really don't talk much at all. Affection stopped a long time ago. Even when we have sex, it's more about just getting off – we don't even kiss anymore. We don't really fight that much – we're just not close. I don't feel like I have a real partner anymore."

## Reality Check

If you believe that love means never arguing, never being hurt, getting all your needs met, sharing the same interests, always being understood, and continually feeling hot for each other, you're headed for major disappointment, discouragement, and heartache. The same is true if you believe that real love doesn't require any work to sustain it. It's important to bring realistic expectations to your relationship and to understand that loving another human being – really loving them – is the most difficult thing you'll ever do. With that understanding, you'll be prepared to invest what it takes to make your relationship a good one. Love as a feeling, as in "falling in love", is effortless. Love as a verb, however, demands that you challenge your self-centeredness and make your partner's needs and wants as important to you as your own. This isn't always easy because your partner experiences the world very differently than you do – even when you believe your partner is your "soul mate".

Accepting that disappointments and disagreements are a normal part of every relationship is a major stress reliever. When you label a situation as a *problem*, you automatically create a stressor and generate a negative reality. Having reasonable expectations of your relationship will minimize the stress of small grievances and decrease the chances of over-reactivity. Connection is then more easily maintained, and your sexual relationship is protected from the impact of petty differences.

## Child-Focused Living

With the celebration of youth and the crumbling of the old hierarchical order of the 50's, children have assumed center stage in the family structure. Family life now revolves around children and their seemingly endless schedule of organized activities – from play groups and t-ball games to piano lessons and cheerleading practice. Family dinners take a back seat to softball practices, and dinner is a quick stop at the McDonald's drive-thru. After practices and dinner, exhausted parents supervise homework sessions and engage in bedtime routines. When the lights finally go out, sex frequently takes a back seat to sleep.

Did any of you grow up this way? In my family, we had dinner every night – around the table – at 6:00 p.m., which coincided with my dad's return home from work. My piano lessons and my brothers' Boy Scout meetings were worked around the family dinner. Homework was our responsibility, and unless it was the dreaded annual science fair project, I don't remember much parental involvement. My parents were nurturing and attentive, but were not tyrannized by an ever-escalating list of child priorities. Family life was busy, but keeping up with it didn't require an Excel spread sheet.

The modern family is complex. At the same time that children took their place in the center of the family, families began facing new economic challenges that created pressure for additional income. Some women were pushed into the workplace, while others happily fled the nest to use their talents outside the home. The end result was an explosion of two income families and increasingly less time to meet the modern child's agenda. Even more time-challenged were the single parents whose numbers jumped considerably during the 70's.

Despite having less time, a University of Maryland study found that today's mothers spend more hours focused on their children than the mothers of the 50's and 60's. In an article from *The Washington Post*, Donna St. George summarized the results of the study which analyzed detailed time diaries kept by thousands of Americans. The number of hours invested by mothers in the direct care of their children jumped from 10.2 hours a week in 1965 to 14.1 hours a week today. And yet, today's mothers still express guilt about not having enough time with their children. Fathers, too, turned more of their attention toward their children, almost tripling their child-focused hours over the last 40 years. With more obligations and an expanded sense of parental responsibility, it's no small wonder that couples are struggling to find their lost desire.

I often hear from beleaguered parents who still wonder if they're giving enough. One father put it this way:

> "My father was never around when I was growing up – he was always at work or down in the basement messing around with different projects – and I swore when I was a dad, I would spend time with my kids. But between work and stuff I have to do around the house, there never seems to be enough time. I go to all my kids' games, I help coach one of their teams, and we have a family outing every Saturday. I also go on one or two field trips each year. My kids don't seem to appreciate it, though. I don't know if I'm not doing enough or if I've done *too* much. I can't remember the last time my wife and I just did something by ourselves."

## Bucking the Trend

It's tough to fight cultural forces that empower children to the level of demigods and that exhort parents to sacrifice exorbitant amounts of time, energy, and money to their service. You can begin, however, to set some reasonable limits on the resources you invest in your children. You can challenge the guilt that surfaces when you refuse to host the end-of- the-season pizza party for the YMCA soccer league or decline the request to fund your teenager's Spring Break in the Bahamas. You and your partner can take that trip to the Bahamas instead. You can organize carpools to reduce the time spent ferrying children to team practices. You can secretly blackmail the coach who plans more than one softball practice a week. You can expect your children to contribute to the upkeep of the household, and you can go on strike until they do.

Janice began making some changes after the last family blow-up:

> "The final straw for me was when my 14-year-old daughter threw a temper tantrum when I refused to cancel my dinner plans with a co-worker to take her and her friends to a movie. There wasn't really anything unusual about her tirade – her typical response to hearing 'no' to anything she wanted was to stomp around the house and slam doors. Something about this time, though, made me see how often we catered to her wants – to all the kids' wants –and how crazy it all was. I knew I was going to be in for some rough times ahead, but I decided right then and there that I was done letting the kids completely run our lives."

I'm not suggesting a return to the days when children were 'seen and not heard'. I am suggesting some reasonableness in negotiating adult needs and child needs. By modeling a healthy respect for your own needs and making both individual and couple time a priority, you teach your children the importance of balance. You also give your children the freedom to define and live their own lives. Most importantly, you eke out a little space and time for re-invigorating your sex life.

## Multi-tasking – Solution or Problem?

Because of the onslaught of demands from children, partners, aging parents, and careers, multi-tasking has surfaced as a popular strategy for jamming everything into the schedule. "Multi-tasking" became the buzz phrase of the 90's. Not surprisingly, between 1965 and 2005 the number of multi-tasking hours has nearly doubled. The model for successful living has become the man or woman who can read emails, provide last minute help with homework, and floss – all while driving the kids to school. Sometimes balls are dropped, like forgetting to pick up a child from Girl Scout Camp, but putting a ball or two down doesn't feel like an option.

The toll of multi-tasking remains hidden and unacknowledged – a bone-weary and mind-numbing fatigue. Overwhelmed by an expanding to-do list and shrinking shut-eye, it's no wonder that sex gets left off of a lot of people's lists. Marcia, a mother of a 12-year-old and a 16-year old, sounded wistful as she described the dwindling frequency of sexual encounters with her husband:

> "Sex was really nice in the beginning. We both had a lot of sexual energy and it wasn't unusual for us to have sex 3-4 times a week. But now, with both of us working and trying to keep up with the kids' activities – it just feels like there's no room for sex in the current scheme of things. We're

lucky now to have sex once or twice a month."

When you're suffering from multi-tasking burn-out and you're operating on a chronic sleep deficit, sex becomes a low priority. You probably don't even care that it's been two months since your last sexual encounter. But although the lack of action may not be of concern to you, it might be to your partner, which in turn creates more stress. Sex often becomes just one more demand among a sea of obligations. It's pretty hard to get in the mood when you're tired, you're mentally rehearsing tomorrow's presentation, and sex feels so much less desirable than the sleep that would help you get through one more day. People who work, raise children, serve on boards, take care of the house, and care for elderly parents may trace the beginning of their sexual shutdown to the stress-filled years when sleep trumped sex. And when you get used to going without, you may stop missing it altogether.

## Mindfulness

The Zen tradition of mindfulness takes multi-tasking to the mat and challenges the notion that the well-lived life is the one that packs the most in. When you squeeze increasingly more tasks and activities into your day, you diminish the presence you bring to your life. You're there, but *you* are not there. Awareness is dulled, and pleasure becomes something scheduled and episodic. On the other hand, doing one thing at a time and being fully present in the moment immediately decreases stress and enhances your capacity for infusing pleasure into even the most mundane tasks. There are certainly times when multi-tasking is sensible or even necessary, like keeping an eye on your two-year-old grandchild while tending the steaks on the grill. But to the degree that your attention is divided as you go about living – either between two or more activities or between one activity and a frantic rehearsal of another future activity – you will add stress, fatigue, and numbness to your life.

You can challenge this debilitating lifestyle by experimenting with maintaining a single focus and bringing a fuller awareness to a few of the activities in your day. Talk on the phone to your mother without wiping down the counters and cabinets; watch a movie without answering emails; sit and enjoy some of your favorite music without just using it as background; challenge yourself to go a full week without talking on your cell phone while driving; stop what you're doing and make full eye contact with your partner when they're talking. Work toward filling your day with the small moments of pleasure that come when you are present in the moment.

**Getting In Charge of Stress**

Stress has the capacity to shut down your sex life. Stress results not only from excessive demands on your time and energy, but from a lack of control, as well. One of the keys to managing stress is to identify where your control lies, and then take charge of what is within your power to control.

First, you exercise control by making whatever changes you can to reduce or eliminate the sources of stress in your life. Setting limits, learning to say no, eliminating those activities that are non-essential and unrewarding, asking for help, hiring help, changing jobs, or changing routines are all examples of using what control you have to de-stress your life. It might be as simple as getting up 15 minutes earlier in the morning to create a less stressful start to the day.

Second, you increase your resistance to stress through better self care and better use of your support system. You know the drill on self care – getting 7-8 hours of sleep each night, exercising 3-4 times a week, eating a healthy diet, taking regular timeouts for fun, remembering to breathe deeply, and laughing on a regular basis. You may be waiting for the day when you'll have more *time* to take care of yourself, but by not making self care a priority, you put yourself at risk for cutting your time even shorter. By failing to attend to the basics of good self-maintenance, you put yourself at risk for illness, depression, or general malaise. Without proper care, your body is ill-equipped to deal long term with the daily onslaught of stress.

You'll also feel the impact of stress far less if you have a support network. Operating in isolation not only limits how much help is available for accomplishing the multitude of tasks facing you each day, it also limits your access to emotional support. That support can make a huge difference when you're going through a particularly stressful time. You need people around you who are caring, empathetic, encouraging, and validating. If that doesn't describe the people in your life, you might want to begin seeking out some new relationships.

The third key to getting in charge of your stress is to remember that you always have control of your response to any given situation.

Changing your perceptions, thoughts, and beliefs about stressors in your life can have a profound effect on the amount of stress they generate, and it's probably one of your least utilized resources. How does this work? You first begin to identify the negative statements and stories that you produce internally during stress and replace that negative internal dialogue with a solution-oriented one. For example, what happens when you say to yourself, "I'm overwhelmed"? You feel further demoralized rather than empowered. This is just one of the many things you may tell yourself that actually helps maintain a high level of stress. You can replace these demoralizing thoughts with more solution-oriented statements. "There's just never enough hours in the day" becomes "I'll find time today for what's most important, and the rest will wait". You begin to recognize your limits, stop catastrophizing, and decide how you want to respond to a given situation. Whether it's a traffic jam, another deadline at work, or a parent who's just been hospitalized, you're in control of how you define the problem and how you talk to yourself about it.

The last important element to changing your response to a stressor over which you have no control is to become less identified with the stressor or the problem. A serious problem commands your attention and often captures you in a feeling of anxiety. But even though you frequently have no control over the outcome, you may find yourself maintaining an obsessive focus on the problem until your life is defined by it. You shrink your focus of attention to the point that you feel cut off from the rest of the world. You no longer have the problem – the problem has you! You loosen its stranglehold grip when you recognize your power to step out of the spell cast by the problem.

In claiming the freedom to determine your response to whatever is wrong in your life, you are empowering yourself to be more than your life circumstances. You're then free to create the life that you want. Hopefully, the life you want is one that includes rich and soul-satisfying sex.

## Final Thoughts

Though we live in a culture that offers a multitude of choices in how we allocate our time and energy, a great many people feel oppressed by those choices rather than liberated by them. We often feel like we're not *choosing* at all. When your weekend is overrun with ferrying children to karate and drum lessons, fixing the broken toilet, grocery shopping, and yard work, there's a sense of victimization rather than freedom. Even when a few hours show up that aren't spoken for, we quickly fill them up with another 'necessary' task, or we collapse in front of the TV for some much-deserved recuperation. Feeling stressed, tired, and always pushed for time puts a great strain on relationships and an even greater strain on sexual desire. When we don't carefully allocate our personal resources, our relationships often end up with just the leftovers, which opens the door for resentment. Investing quality time and energy in your partner and in your sexual relationship is an important step in taking sexy back.

## *Exercise*

Take some time to think about possible factors impacting your sexual desire. After each item that you check, jot down some thoughts about how you've been affected and how you feel about it.

☐ Child Focus_____

_____

_____

_____

☐ Relationship Issues_____

_____

_____

_____

☐ Multi-tasking_____

_____

_____

_____

☐ Stress_____

_____

_____

_____

☐ Others_____

_____

_____

_____

# Chapter 7

## Resentment: #1 Enemy of Desire

Resentment is the slow, simmering, seething anger that gradually destroys the foundation of a relationship. Like termites, resentment does its dirty work behind the scenes, relatively unnoticed. Sadly, just as a termite-infested house may remain standing as inner structures crumble, the relationship may endure as resentment slowly kills off desire bit-by-bit. How much desire are you going to feel for the partner who recklessly spends more than your joint incomes, sabotages your authority with the kids, or makes snide comments about your weight?

Judy came to me at her husband, Ken's urging because their sex life was practically non-existent. She hadn't felt any sexual desire for over a year and was at a loss to explain why, especially since she still loved her husband. She went to the doctor and didn't find any physical explanation. Judy felt terrible about her husband's unhappiness, and she desperately wanted to feel physical passion for him again. In the early years of their marriage, Judy was a full-time mom and homemaker. Ken had become accustomed to doing little more around the house than cutting the grass in the summer. Two years ago, however, Judy returned to her career as an accountant, often working 50-60 hours a week during tax season. But – you guessed it – she continued to carry full responsibility for running the household. Old habits die hard, and despite her pleas for help, Ken never really stepped up to the plate to assume a more equitable share of the chores. Oh, sometimes he would run the sweeper when asked, and every couple of months he would clean his bathroom, but mostly he just seemed to tune out Judy's requests and complaints. Judy usually did everything in her power to avoid conflict, so although her resentment was building, there wasn't much fighting in the marriage. What their relationship did suffer from was a gradually accumulating resentment that eventually shut down Judy's sexual desire.

The familiar story of women carrying a disproportionate share of household responsibilities feels tired and trite. But it's a story I hear almost daily from clients, friends, and acquaintances, and one that is backed up by virtually every survey conducted on household division of labor. It's little wonder that the woman who falls exhausted into bed on Sunday night after an endless round of errands and household chores is not responsive to the come-ons of the partner she watched lying on the couch all afternoon engrossed in a football game. She may not connect her lack of sexual interest with her anger about assuming responsibility for more than her fair share, but the sense of unfairness she feels often leaves her stewing in some angry juices. Despite the feminist movement and men's increasing willingness to load the dishwasher and mop the kitchen floor, an inequitable division of labor remains a huge source of resentment in many marriages.

## Unexpressed Anger

Anger turns into resentment when it goes unexpressed. Many people are conflict-avoidant and will do almost anything to avoid a fight. When they're unhappy about something in their relationship, they often don't address it directly because they anticipate defensiveness that might lead to conflict. Conflict avoiders may offer subtle hints about a situation they're upset about, or they may use a passive-aggressive approach such as pouting in an effort to get their needs met. They won't, however, just come right out and say, "I'm pissed off that you don't call me when you're going to be late coming home." People who avoid conflict do so for any number of reasons. They may have learned from early experiences that conflict is dangerous and find themselves intimidated by the anger of others. They may fear being unable to hold their own in an argument, or they may not believe that conflict can produce any positive outcomes. They may also fear losing control of their own anger. Whatever the reason, the inability to handle conflict provides a very fertile ground in which resentment can grow.

I've often seen low-conflict relationships go up in smoke when the quiet, easy-going, conflict-avoider wakes up one day and announces to their partner, "I'm not in love with you anymore." Though it may feel to their partner like a bolt out of the blue, the resentment has been silently building for years. And because the person who hates and avoids conflict is also loathe to end a relationship, they will often stay in the relationship until something (and more often, some*one*) provides the necessary push to get out. A person filled with resentment toward their partner is someone who's extremely vulnerable to an affair. A new person with no baggage and fresh promises easily resuscitates desire. That was the story I heard from Maxine:

> "I thought we were happy – I really did. We had the little everyday problems that everyone has, but nothing serious. Paul always told me he loved me and we talked a lot about the future. I never dreamed he was so miserable. Why did he wait until *after* he moved out of the house and started screwing someone else to tell me how he really felt - how he always felt unappreciated and how much he hated it when I yelled. He said he feels dead inside and doesn't think he can ever regain that "in love" feeling for me. This is the man I adored – I would have done anything he asked to make him happy. But he never asked...."

## Stonewalling

Another breeding ground for resentment is when anger *is* expressed but falls on deaf ears. When anger fails to bring about change, resignation often sets in. Even people who are upfront with their partner about hurt and frustration will only continue to express their unhappiness for so long if they're repeatedly met with defensiveness and resistance. They then begin to shut down because of the vulnerability involved in asking for what they want and need. When wants and needs go unfulfilled, it stops feeling safe to ask. The shutdown is a retreat into greater self-protectiveness, and that retreat then translates into less investment in the relationship. There's a general sense of hopelessness and defeat – "she'll never change" – that sets the stage for giving up. Communication breakdown affects both partners because the person who has given up continues building resentment while their mate is left wondering, "what the hell?".

I once heard an interesting description of this phenomenon in a workshop given by Caroline Myss, a medical intuitive and mystic. She said that we all walk through life carrying buckets filled to the brim with pain we've accumulated during our journey. We walk very carefully so that we don't spill a drop. We protect our buckets because if we allow any pain to spill out, there will be room for new pain – and we prefer the familiar to the new. The problem is, if we stay attached to our old pain, we're blocking anything new from happening to us. Our future is simply the past that we throw in front of us and keep replaying – which is hardly a future. Resentment and the unwillingness to take a risk can keep us locked into a life of reruns. Betsy and Tim had more than enough reruns in their 22-year marriage:

"When we finally decided to go to marriage counseling, we were both feeling pretty hopeless about turning things around. We had plenty of anger stored up, and I think each of us was waiting for the other to change first. It was a standoff. In the first couple of sessions, it was like we were competing for who had been short-changed the most in the marriage – hoping that the therapist would make the other one shape up. But of course, that's not what happened. It turns out that the changes we made for each other were not that hard – what was hard was creating a clean slate and believing that the other person could change. I think we both felt safe as long as we were shut down and unhappy. Giving up the anger and the hopelessness was hard, but that's when things really started changing. I still have to catch myself when I notice I'm thinking the changes are only temporary and everything's going to go back to the way it was. I know if I keep thinking that way, I'm starting the reruns all over again."

Stepping out of long-held resentment can be a challenge, and you may need help from a therapist if you find that your best efforts to 'let go' just aren't working. A therapist can help you overcome the obstacles preventing you from resolving resentment. The rest of this chapter addresses how to avoid accumulating new resentment.

## Making Your Relationship Resentment-Proof

### Keep your voice

Don't be afraid to speak up when your feelings are hurt, your needs aren't being met, or you disagree with your partner. Put your wants out on the table, whether it's where to go for dinner or what to do with your tax refund. It's not fair to expect your partner to read your mind, and it's romantic crap to believe that if s/he really loved you, s/he would know what you want. Your partner looks at the world through a different set of lenses that create completely different perceptions and understandings. For example, arriving late to a movie may not be a big deal to you but may be a very big deal to your partner. In relationships, it's not as much about right and wrong nearly as often as it is about differing needs. When Arlene complained to me about her husband, Fred, she clearly thought he was wrong:

> "Every night he stays up watching TV until 1 or 2 in the morning even though I've told him how much I want us to go to bed together. I have to hit the bed by 11 or I'm worthless the next day, but I hate going to bed by myself. What's the point of being married if I'm lying alone in bed every night? I think he loves that damn television more than he loves me!"

Arlene had done a good job of letting her wants be known, but failed to take into account her husband's 'want'. What she didn't understand, because Fred had neglected to tell her, was that the late hours spent watching television helped him relax. Fred had a demanding job dealing with people all day long and relished the alone time after Arlene went to bed. After acknowledging the legitimacy of both their needs, Fred and Arlene were able to work out a compromise – Fred agreed to lie down and cuddle with Arlene from 11:00-11:30 before returning to the family room for his television time.

If you care about your partner, you're obligated to care about what's important to them - even if it seems ridiculous. By the same token, they're obligated to care about what's important to you – which, of course, is never ridiculous! Love grows in an environment where each partner feels like their needs are taken seriously. Successful conflict resolution – and the avoidance of resentment – requires a clear intention to honor the needs of both parties, however imperfectly. Relationships require a lot of compromise and accommodation, which is difficult because in the end, each partner's need may be only partially met. But the resistance to compromise generally reflects discomfort rather a lack of love. You'd probably both like to love each other without ever having to sacrifice anything that you want. Learning where you can give in order to accommodate your partner's differences is one of the challenges of relationships.

## Handling the Small Stuff

The top of the desk in my bedroom hasn't seen the light of day for more years than I want to count. It's covered with stacks of books, magazines, and miscellaneous papers – all belonging to my husband. In *my* comfort zone, there's minimal clutter and desk tops are visible. For several years, I fought this battle with my husband whose best efforts to accommodate my wishes never resulted in more than a slight dent in the mounds of 'stuff'. I finally decided that all this 'stuff', no matter how much space it consumed, was 'small stuff' – not worth my anger, the nagging, or the battles with my husband. Once I accepted this reality, my challenge became how to truly let it go. I began by forcing myself to find something positive in all that clutter. I didn't want to. I wanted my husband to be 'wrong', admit that he was wrong, and do something about it! But after pushing beyond the whole right and wrong dynamic, I realized that those stacks of books and magazines represented something I love about my husband – his passion for learning. He's usually reading several books at one time and is constantly finding articles of interest in National Geographic or in an environmental magazine that he just has to save. Now every time I look at that desk, I think of that positive association and I tell myself that the clutter itself is small potatoes. I still wish he'd develop a filing system – and use it. And I haven't changed my preference for order and clean desk tops, but I've stretched my comfort zone just enough to include a little mess.

Even small stuff, day after day, month after month, can create resentment if it's the kind of crap that really sticks in your craw. Often when you believe you're letting go of anger over something trivial, you're actually just stuffing it in the sack of grievances you'll later use as ammunition during the next argument with your partner. It's sometimes difficult to be honest with yourself about when you're letting go rather than holding on. If you're gritting your teeth and cursing under your breath while refilling the empty towel dispenser – again! – you probably haven't let it go, and it will remain a source of resentment.

Some of the irritating things your partner does only bug you because you do them differently. The arguments about the proper way to load the dishwasher, balance the checkbook, or fold towels, all have to do with wanting things *your way*. The reason these ludicrous arguments can be so intense in a relationship is that couples are really fighting about who holds the power – whose needs are going to get met? When couples come into a marital session reporting a terrible argument in the previous week but neither can remember what it was about, I know that those bigger questions were at play. If you're frequently engaged in a power struggle with your partner, neither of you are going to be very successful in getting your needs met, and both of you are likely to hold the other responsible. That's another breeding ground for resentment.

Only you can decide what you can and can't live with – what's the small stuff and what's the big stuff. Just be sure that you're not putting the entire burden on your partner to change the things you don't like. Start with compromise and see if you can figure out what works for both of you. If you decide to push yourself to make an accommodation, find a way to accommodate without feeling resentful. Do an occasional check on your resentment meter to keep resentment from sneaking in the back door. If you notice some resentment creeping in and you're not successful in getting in charge of it, then it's time to come back to your partner and ask for what you need. Put your need in the form of a request rather than a complaint. Complaints create immediate defensiveness, which decreases the chance that your need is going to be met. Instead of, "I hate it when you leave little blobs of toothpaste in the sink", try "I'd really appreciate it if you'd rinse out the sink after brushing your teeth". And watch your tone...

### You're Not My Parent!!

Do you notice what a trigger it is when your partner scolds, lectures, or nags you? Nobody wants a parent for a partner. But parent-child interactions are a common dynamic in couple relationships and are a major source of resentment. This dynamic is a losing proposition from both sides because the parental position is usually born of frustration, and the child position typically stems from a sense of powerlessness. Both partners can easily justify their parental or child-like behavior by referring to the "controlling" or "irresponsible" behavior of the other. But whether your partner is acting like an obstreperous 10-year-old or doing a good imitation of your dad, it is crucial that you relate to each other as adults.

No lasting solutions come out of parent-child interactions in a couple relationship because the imbalance of power precludes adult cooperation. You may wonder why a partner's child-like behavior should warrant an adult response. Bottom line, your partner isn't going to change the behavior you want changed as long as they're treated like a child. Adults that are treated like children tend to react like children – with rebellion, resistance, and defiance.

Another one of the inane battles my husband and I had in the early years of our marriage erupted every couple of months when my husband would discover, only after getting into the shower and getting soaking wet, that there was only a small sliver of soap left in the soap dish. That meant he had to get out of the shower, drip his way over to the sink, and get out a new bar of soap. After suffering through this terrible ordeal and finishing his shower, he would come looking for me – loaded for bear. I tuned out pretty quickly when he started yelling, but I think his tirade went something like, "Why can't you ever replace the #%*^@ soap in the shower stall when it gets too small to use?? You *never* remember to put in a new bar and then I have to get out of the shower..." You get the drift. My response was usually at the same decibel level and went something like, "I didn't know I was the keeper of the soap. You're an adult – you can look in the shower before you get in and make sure there's a usable bar of soap....blah, blah, blah." Not once after any of those yelling matches did I feel the least bit inclined to change my behavior and do what my husband wanted. I felt like a child being scolded by an angry parent, and I wasn't about to comply with his demands. Maybe I'm more rebellious than most, but I don't think my response was so unusual. I didn't change my behavior until the day when my husband calmly explained how much it meant to him when I anticipated his forgetfulness and his need – and replaced the shower soap. Knowing that I valued his need – no matter how silly or trivial – made him feel loved. That was a light bulb moment for me – noticing how different it felt to consider doing something out of love rather than out of compliance.

Even if you're less rebellious than I am and manage to change your behavior to comply with your partner's demands (or to avoid their anger), you're likely to build resentment in the process. Avoid this resentment by not responding from the child position with either rebellion or compliance. And be sure your children are the only family members you're parenting.

## Try Something Different

Taking a different approach with your partner can make a huge difference in how they respond to you. You've probably heard all of your life that you can't change another person – you can only change yourself. What that little piece of conventional wisdom fails to recognize is that if you accomplish the latter, you'll accomplish the former. Because you and your partner are connected and part of a system, change on your part invites change from your partner. If your partner hasn't responded to your attempts to get them to change, don't assume that it can't or won't happen. Maybe you need to be less critical – maybe you need to step out of the parental role – maybe you need a softer startup – or maybe you need outside intervention. Change is difficult, and it's human nature to resist it. But with the right motivation, it's certainly possible – even when it's only one of you who's trying.

## Do What You Want

Don't do things you really don't want to do. At this point, you're probably thinking I'm from another planet – you know, that alternate universe where your every wish is magically fulfilled and everyone else exists only for the purpose of serving you. But hear me out. At any given moment in time, you have multiple needs and wants – some of which are in conflict. Maybe you woke up this morning and your first coherent thought was, "I don't want to get up and go to work." The 'want' to stay in bed is the one that feels the most pressing – the one that you can most easily identify. But underneath that want are other wants – like you want to be responsible, you want to earn money, you want a promotion, you want to be dependable, or you want to keep your lunch date with a friend. If you don't take a moment to get in touch with those other wants, you'll either follow your first want and stay in bed, or, in a more likely scenario, you'll drag yourself out of bed after hitting the snooze button four times and feel resentful that you're doing something you don't want to do. Again. It's a good way to go through life as a victim.

I first began to clarify my wants more diligently when my children were young and I was working full-time. In those days, I frequently found myself doing things for the kids that I didn't 'want' to do, and I was building up resentment in the process. I didn't want to resent being a mother, and I certainly didn't want to resent my kids, so I began to identify the 'wants' that were underneath the 'don't wants'. If it was a T-ball game I didn't want to attend, I'd think about wanting to watch my child digging in the dirt in the outfield or running the bases after finally connecting with the ball. I'd think about just wanting to be a part of my child's life, or I'd think about the bratwurst I could get at the concession stand. Whatever it took, I either identified the wants underneath the "don't want" or I gave myself permission not to go to the game. That's what I want for you. Either decide that you *want* to do something or don't do it. If I'm ironing all my husband's shirts and despising every minute of it, I'm likely to begin resenting the wearer of the shirts even if it's my decision to iron (fat chance) rather than a expectation from my husband. I can decide I want to do it because it's a loving thing to do for my partner or because I like the way he looks in nicely ironed shirts, or I can explore other options: teach my husband how to iron his own shirts, send them out to the laundry, or my personal favorite, take the damp shirts out of the dryer and hang them to dry. Giving myself options helps avoid the possible build-up of resentment.

## Pay Attention

A neglected relationship is fertile ground in which resentment can grow. It's important to make your relationship a priority and carve out couple time regardless of the obstacles. Do one thing every day that injects positive energy into the relationship even if that one thing is just a moment of reflection on one of your partner's better qualities. Don't let distance grow between you. Resentment can create distance, but if you and your partner have just gradually grown apart over time, it's easy to resent things that you might more easily accept if you were close. Attention paid to your partner is like a deposit in the emotional bank account of your relationship. The inevitable small irritations and disappointments with your partner that are withdrawals from that account are more easily forgiven when the account is in the black.

## Be a Positive Storyteller

Watch the stories you tell yourself about your partner's behavior. We are constantly interpreting and assigning particular meaning to everything that happens to us. The problem is that we often forget that our interpretation is not the 'truth', but an assessment based on how we experience the world and how we're feeling at the time. If a husband is angry with his wife, he's much more likely to assign negative meaning to her behavior than if he's not angry. Let's take a small sample of behavior experienced from two different emotional states:

Jim stays home sick from work. He calls his wife and asks her to stop off at the drugstore on her way home to pick up a prescription for him. She arrives home a couple of hours later – sans the prescription. She's apologetic – she simply forgot.

The story Jim tells himself about his wife's forgetfulness – and how he responds to her – will be influenced by how connected they are, how he's feeling toward her, and how much is in their emotional bank account. From an angry, disconnected place, Jim tells himself a story about his wife's self-centeredness, her lack of caring, her complete disregard for his needs, and her overall unfitness for the human race. From a loving, connected place, Jim tells himself a story about his wife as a distracted and very busy woman who really does care about him, who feels terrible about forgetting the prescription, and who will gladly go back out to get it. It's the same event but two very different stories about what that event means. Neither story represents absolute truth, but the second story creates a lot less anger, hurt, and resentment – for both parties.

If you want to avoid accumulating resentment in your relationship, it's important to be generous with the stories you tell yourself about your partner, especially in regard to sex. You owe it to yourself to try on stories that point to solutions rather than flood you with hopelessness and that create connections rather than distance. Give your partner every benefit of the doubt and every chance to be interpreted through the lens of love. That lens is incredibly forgiving and prevents resentment from growing. Without resentment, you can tell a story that empowers you to be as passionate, as engaged, and as sexy as you want to be.

## Stay in Touch

It's more difficult for resentment to build when you maintain physical affection and an active sex life. As we've seen, resentment, alone, can squash desire very quickly, but rejection between the sheets can produce its own hard feelings. A negative cycle can ensue in which both partners are resentful – for different reasons – and sex becomes about as likely as both partners taking ownership for their role in the drama. The hormones and neurotransmitters released during sex create connection, trust, and intimacy, which together produce a pretty potent vaccine against resentment. Just as it's critical to avoid resentment if you want a healthy sex life, it's critical to have a healthy sex life in order to avoid building resentment.

## Do Monthly Check-Ups

Schedule a regular monthly 'check-up' for your relationship in which you ask yourself and then your partner what's working and what's problematic in your life together. Make it a time of mutual problem-solving over a glass of wine. Avoid the attack and counter-attack moves that are part of the blaming scenario in so many relationships. If you can't manage these check-ups on your own, then schedule a monthly meeting with a couple's therapist. It will be the best investment you can make in your relationship – and a lot cheaper than divorce.

Seeking out the help of a therapist is also recommended if you're struggling with resentment that is related to your partner's infidelity. Infidelity wreaks havoc with the trust and safety that are so necessary for physical intimacy to flourish. It *is* possible to heal the wounds created by a partner's affair, but it takes time and often requires professional help.

## De-Mythologize Love

Many of my clients ask me if it's possible to feel 'in love' again with a partner who long ago ceased to stir those emotions. This question reflects the romantic myth of love as a magical spell that is mysteriously cast upon a lover and their beloved – a spell that once broken, is impossible to recapture. Certainly being in the throes of romantic love can feel like a spell since it's accompanied by a surge in hormones and the release of feel-good chemicals in the brain. But unfortunately, this euphoric state of oneness is only temporary – gradually fading when the different worldviews of each partner begin colliding. That's when the messy business of real love begins. Forced to face our separateness and our differences, it becomes a challenge to maintain our passion and our desire for the partner who once felt impossible to resist. It's easier to 'fall in love' with someone new, except that the new love will eventually fall victim to the same disillusionment. It's absolutely possible to feel 'in love' with your current partner again if you can leave the past behind and are willing to risk vulnerability. Finding new ways of meeting each other's needs and accepting each other's differences may be a lot more work than magic, but it's the only formula we have for making love last.

## Final Thoughts

Tending to a relationship is much like caring for a garden. There's planting what you want to grow, nurturing and protecting all that you value, and carefully watching and weeding out the undesirable. It involves a major investment of time and energy. Relationships that are victims of benign neglect resemble a garden that has become overgrown and choked with weeds. When couples allow resentment to grow unchecked, it will take over the relationship and strangle the life out of all that is tender and beautiful between them. The writer, Malachy McCourt, once said, "Resentment is like taking poison and waiting for the other person to die". Keeping a check on resentment is critical to the survival of a relationship – and even more critical to maintaining passion and desire.

# Exercise

Use the following questions to help you assess your risk for accumulating resentment in your relationship.

1. When I know that something I want to say or do might cause conflict with my partner, I

    a. go ahead with it and deal with any conflict that comes up
    b. wait until my partner is in a good mood and then approach it very gingerly
    c. try to figure out how to get what I want without approaching my partner
    d. probably would just forget about it – it's not worth a fight

2. When I'm angry with my partner, I

    a. go for it full throttle
    b. try to share my anger without attacking
    c. pout or do the old 'silent treatment'
    d. keep it to myself

3. When I've expressed anger to my partner, but nothing ever changes, I

    a. have a serious sit-down with my partner and make sure that I don't leave without a commitment for change
    b. try changing how I deliver the message
    c. find some other ways of getting my needs met
    d. give up – it's not worth it

4. When it comes to speaking up about what I want, I

    a. put it right out there
    b. state my preference but make it clear I'm willing to compromise
    c. provide lots of hints but don't come right out with it
    d. pretty much keep it to myself and hope my partner figures it out

5. When I find myself feeling irritated by small stuff in my relationship, I

    a. talk to my partner about it or find a way of letting it go
    b. let it build until it becomes big stuff – then deal with it
    c. shut down until my partner asks me what is wrong
    d. keep it to myself and just learn to live with it

6. When my partner fails to meet a need that I've verbalized, I

    a. schedule a time to talk about what's getting in the way
    b. get mad and raise a ruckus
    c. feel hurt that my need doesn't seem to matter
    d. assume that my partner is selfish and unwilling to do what I've asked

7. I'm guilty of acting like a parent with my partner or responding like a child

    a. rarely
    b. sometimes
    c. frequently
    d. I don't know any other way to be

8. When I think about what changes I'd like to see in my relationship, I

    a. try to figure out what I could do differently to make them happen

    b. try to figure out how to get my partner on board

    c. feel pessimistic and end up trying to be okay with things not changing

    d. feel hopeless that things will ever change and do nothing

9. When I look at how I live my life, I

    a. do a pretty good job of staying aware of my choices and do what I want to do

    b. do a lot of things I want to do, but also put a lot of effort into being what other other people need me to be

    c. often give up what I want because there's so much that I have to do

    d. never even stop to think about what I want

10. When I talk to myself about things my partner does that disappoint me, I

    a. try to see it from my partner's side and give the benefit of the doubt

    b. remind myself that disappointment is a part of every relationship

    c. try not to get too bent out of shape over it

    d. have a hard time not focusing on my partner's selfishness

# Chapter 8

## Sex Talk: Was It Good for You?

A recent headline in the *New York Times* read, "Children's book creates a furor with one word". The book, *The Higher Power of Lucky*, was none other than the 2007 winner of the Newbery Medal, and the firestorm of criticism was ignited over the use of the word "scrotum" on the opening page. Not even a human scrotum, but a dog's scrotum! – as in a rattlesnake bit the dog on the scrotum. Great concern was expressed over the appropriateness of including such a word in a book intended for 9 to 12 year olds. Do the censors think that 'scrotum' is sexually stimulating? Dirty? Corrupting? I don't really know what goes through a prepubescent mind after stumbling across the word 'scrotum' in a story, but I seriously doubt that it's a turning point toward perversity. The truth is that the very censorship designed to 'protect' children has created a society of sexual mutes.

People may be having sex, but most of them are not talking about it. Many people would rather have bad sex or no sex at all than have an open, straightforward conversation about sex.

Of course, people do talk about sex, but the talk is heavy on jokes, innuendo, conquests, and complaints. Healthy dialogue about sexuality is virtually absent, particularly in couple relationships. You might confide sexual secrets to your best friend, your sister, or a stranger on the internet but choke when it comes to sharing sexual preferences with your partner. Even those of you who are generally pretty open about sex may find talking about it with your partner highly uncomfortable.

It's amazing that we aren't all natural sex-talkers given our exposure to sexual imagery and sexual language. From beer commercials featuring bouncing bikini-clad blondes to *Cosmo* covers promising "Ten Secret Tips for Five-Minute Orgasms", the public face of sexuality is anything but shy. But squeamishness and sensationalism often go hand-in-hand in a society that can't seem to make up its mind about sex. Growing up in America, we're dished a healthy portion of shame along side the Victoria's Secret models, *Playboy* magazines, and Desperate Housewives.

**Sexual Silence**

You probably grew up in a family where there was no sex – at least none that anyone was talking about. The private parts of your body were so private they had secret code names like pocketbook or tallywhacker. You learned a lot from the secrecy and the silence – it spoke volumes. Though children have to be socialized in respect to the private parts of their bodies, shame has unfortunately become the default teaching tool for that socialization. Shame may be used for teaching table manners, too, but there's an intensity connected to reprimands about playing with your pecker or pookie that leaves an indelible mark. I rarely hear stories of adults traumatized by being told not to play with their food.

In my years as a sex educator, I often heard teenage girls refer to their genitals as "down there". When I explained to them how diaphragms were inserted to prevent pregnancy, I got comments like, "You mean I have to touch myself *down there?*" These children of 70's feminists, the same feminists who urged women to look at their genitals with hand mirrors, were repulsed by the idea of that much familiarity with their vaginas. Eventually it stopped surprising me when I had to define the function of the clitoris or explain that the correct term for a female's external genitalia was vulva rather than vagina.

Without a model for healthy sexual dialogue, an attempt at sexual conversation can be like assembling an Ikea entertainment center without instructions. Bullied by awkwardness and fear, many just avoid that conversation altogether. I see couples in my office who have shared bathrooms and have swapped bodily fluids for years but have never had sex talk beyond, "Do you wanna go to bed early tonight?" Sex is both simple and enormously complex. Anybody can put a peg in a hole, so to speak, but the challenge of meshing unique sexual histories, desires, and responses is quite another matter. Anything more than a one-night stand is going to take some conversation.

Sex holds the power to wound and heal, divide and unite. Couples are more likely to harness the healing and bonding power of sex when they are willing to keep talking despite the anxiety and clumsiness of sex talk. Tammy, a client whose husband resisted her previous attempts to talk about sex, finally stood up to his resistance and plowed forward:

> "I used to shut down and walk away discouraged when he didn't want to talk, but after years of anger and disappointment, I decided to let him know how I felt. Sex was impersonal, and I just didn't feel anything anymore. First, he rolled his eyes, as usual. This time I ignored it and told him I wanted to make sex better for him and for me. He seemed unsure of exactly where I was headed, but he could tell I was serious and at least started paying attention."

After deciding to take the plunge, you may find yourself lacking a comfortable sexual vocabulary. The words, themselves, can be another barrier to sex talk.

### Dirty Words

It's a helluva choice between fellatio and 'blowjob' or cunnilingus and 'eating out'. Penis sounds diminutive somehow but 'dick' and 'cock' seem better suited to lustful whispers in the bedroom than to a conversation at the kitchen table over coffee.

Women's genitalia are even worse. 'Pussy' just feels wrong unless it's uttered in the heat of passion, but who wants to talk about the vulva, the labia, or the vagina? 'Making love' is an attempt at something between 'fucking' and intercourse, but many sexual acts and body parts lack that softer vocabulary. What we need is a soft, sexy set of words. We need words that aren't used as curses and angry insults but convey more than the clinical terminology found in biology textbooks.

What's with the insults? Have you ever thought about how your sexuality has been warped by the use of sexual language to express road rage or trash talk the opposing team? Think about what the phrases 'fuck off', 'fucked up' and 'fuck it' say about our views on 'fucking'. We have lots of angry expressions that refer to oral sex: 'cocksucker', 'cock breath', 'blow me', 'eat me', 'suck it'. Why use such a popular activity to express contempt? Even the slang terms for male and female genitals – 'dick', 'dickhead', 'pussy', 'twat' – are used to insult and injure. No wonder we have a language problem when it comes to talking about sex!

Even without the angry associations, slang may be way outside your comfort zone. The proper names, however, don't exactly roll off the tongue. Experiment until you find the language that's comfortable for you and your partner. Share which words are 'hot' words for you and which ones leave you cold. Together you can make up your own words and develop a unique love language. The writer/producer of the series,

"Grey's Anatomy", complained that the network objected to her using the word 'vagina' too much in the show. So one of the show's assistants came up with the word 'va-jay-jay' to use in place of vagina. Interestingly enough, there was not a similar objection to the use of the word 'penis'.

You may want two sets of language – one for conversational use and one for lovemaking. Words and phrases that can be a turn-off outside the bedroom can be a real turn-on in the heat of passion. Just be sure that you and your partner are on the same page with the language you use. The 'Dirty Word Game' at the end of the chapter can help you come up with a common language.

Once you decide on a language to use, you may still need practice to get comfortable with saying the words aloud. A colleague once asked me how to get comfortable with using sexual terminology in front of an audience. She was starting to teach sex education classes in her high school and wanted to feel at ease in talking with the students. I advised her to stand in front of a mirror and practice saying penis, testicles, vulva, and vagina over and over until it no longer felt like she was coughing up a hairball.

## Vulnerability

Fred asked for my help in talking to his wife, Susan, about certain aspects of their lovemaking. The couple had a good relationship and both enjoyed having sex. Fred was a big fan of oral sex, and Susan had no problem with including it as part of their sexual repertoire. However, when Fred tried to tell Susan exactly how he liked to be orally stimulated, Susan became irate and said, "If you don't like the way I do it, then I just won't do it at all! Most men would be happy to get head, period!" Fred hadn't meant to be critical and actually thought Susan would welcome tips on how to give him the most pleasure. But Fred's 'instructions' made Susan feel inadequate and spoiled her enjoyment of the act.

Most people are highly sensitive to even the slightest hint of criticism when it comes to their sexuality or sexual performance. I mean, how many really acceptable answers are there to the question, "Was it good for you?" Lovers are also very reluctant to put their partner in the position of getting feedback that they, themselves, might want to avoid. It's kind of a mutual protection pact: I won't say anything to you if you don't say anything to me. Unfortunately, the pact may shut down all sexual feedback. You might fear that if you tell your partner what you'd like for them to do, you may get a negative response. They might feel badly that they weren't already doing what you suggested or feel criticized for what they were doing instead. Or, like Susan, they may even take offense at needing 'instructions' at all!

Sensitive sexual egos need protection, but not silence. By carefully choosing words that are encouraging and positive, you respect your partner's vulnerability and communicate an interest in improving your sexual relationship. The timing of feedback is also important. Right in the middle of sex is not the time to tell your partner that you hate the way he grabs your va-jay-jay. However, you can share how-to tips during specific times of sexual exploration, with you and your partner taking turns as 'instructor'. Otherwise, feedback can wait until another time when you are both relaxed, well fed, and feeling connected to one another.

## Getting Defensive

Susan responded to Fred with defensiveness. Many couples have not learned how to discuss sensitive topics such as in-laws, money, or sex without triggering an immediate and predictable defensive response. Insecurity and a need to preserve your worldview often result in resistance to new input. Change is scary. Letting in your partner's perspective can take you outside of your comfort zone. Maintaining a defensive position is an attempt to stay inside that zone but eliminates the opportunity for discussion, compromise, and growth.

Defensiveness quickly escalates a 'discussion' into a heated argument. When you become defensive, you stop hearing your partner and dialogue shuts down. You really stop *wanting* to hear your partner. All of your energy is focused on self-protection rather than trying to understand what your partner is saying. But talking about sex doesn't have to trigger negativity. Though you don't have complete control over your partner's reaction, you can minimize the risk of a defensive response by picking the right time and place for a discussion, using a gentle startup, and avoiding critical language.

## Getting Un-defensive

A gentle startup is important to keeping a dialogue open and productive. "You're bad at..." or "Can you please stop..." probably won't get the response you're looking for. Avoid beginning with a complaint. Start your sentences with "I" instead of "you", and avoid the words "always" and "never". It's also imperative that you focus more on what you like rather than what you don't like. For example, "The thing that turns me on the most is..." or "I really love it when you...". When there's a need to share information about something you dislike, avoid being critical. Try, "For some reason, I tense up when..." or "I just have a thing about...". Then it's more about you than about your partner.

Tell your partner that you value your sexual relationship and that you want to be able to talk about it. Acknowledge any anxiety you're feeling in bringing it up and ask for help in dealing with the anxiety. Explain how important it is for you to be able to talk about sex without it becoming an argument. Stress the need for both of you to stay calm and avoid sarcasm or criticism. Ask your partner to let you know if they start feeling defensive, and commit to steering the conversation in a more positive direction if that occurs. Be willing to postpone the talk for another time if you get caught in a negative loop.

For the last few months, Kelly found herself making one excuse after another when John tried to initiate sex. She felt guilty about avoiding sex and finally decided to break the tension that had developed in the relationship by starting a different kind of dialogue.

> "I know I haven't been into sex lately, and I feel really bad about it. I just never think about it, and it's not easy for me to get myself in the mood. It's not about you. For some reason, I just don't have any sex drive these days. I wanna work on it. It's important to me. But I hope you can understand where I am and be patient."

Because John didn't feel attacked, he didn't get defensive and was actually able to join Kelly in brainstorming some solutions for improving their sex life.

**Fabio is a Fake**

A female client complained to me about her partner's "constant need to talk" when they were being intimate. As she put it, "Maybe I've just read too many romance novels, but it kind of spoils it for me when he's always saying, "how does that feel?" or "do you like that?" when we're in the middle of making love. The men in the novels just know what to do – they don't have to ask. Giving directions during sex is like getting a massage and having to tell the masseuse how to do her job."

People sometimes suffer under the illusion that sex is natural and you shouldn't have to talk about it. This belief is part of the romantic myth that two people who love each other will automatically know how to please each other sexually. However, each person's unique sexual response map is learned only through sensitive touch and verbal sharing. It's unrealistic to expect your partner to intuit your needs and wants in the sexual arena. Did you expect your partner to automatically 'know' about your passion for hotel bar karaoke or your hatred for noodles in your chili? Your partner comes to know you through the communication of your likes and dislikes. The wants and needs in your physical relationship are no exception. If giving feedback during sex is a distraction and a turn-off, then find another time to talk. Unless your partner is a gifted clairvoyant, your chances for good sex will certainly improve if you learn to talk about it.

### "Hey, Baby….." What's There to Talk About?

Okay – You've come up with a comfortable sexual language, you feel safe enough to risk being vulnerable, and you're working on keeping defensiveness to a minimum. Now here are a few discussion topics to get you started on a sexual dialogue. The goal is to abandon your pact of silence and create an openness that will facilitate a discussion of sexual feelings, thoughts, and preferences.

## In General

Share how you feel about the sex in your relationship. Is it a source of conflict? Does it bring you closer? Discuss what you like the most about your sex together. Talk about how your sexual relationship has changed over time. Reminisce about favorite sexual memories. Describe what you 'get' from sex and why it's important to you. Share your vision of the ideal sexual relationship.

## The Start-Up

Part of creating more passion is learning to play with gestures, facial expressions, and body language. It's the art of flirtation and seduction. Couples make a big mistake when they stop flirting with each other when the courtship is over. Flirting makes your partner feel wanted, valued, and desired. If your seduction skills have become a bit rusty, try reviving them on your next date night. Look directly into your partner's eyes, let your hand barely graze her thigh, breathe softly into his ear during a slow dance. It's all coming back to you, right?

And then there's the life where you live the other 98% of the time – the life that includes the screaming match with your 15-year-old, the mess to clean up in the basement, and the next day's soccer tournament. Though seduction is terrific in reviving passion, it's just not going to happen on a routine basis. That's why it's important to discuss how you want to let each other know when you're interested in sex.

I hear women complain about being grabbed in the crotch, humped from behind, flashed, or crudely propositioned when their partner wants some action. That kind of approach is unlikely to elicit a ye-ha from a low desire woman. I also hear from men who resent the expectation to 'perform' at the first hint of sexual interest from their partner, regardless of their frame of mind, fatigue level, or what playoff game is on TV.

Initiating sex is risky business. Hearing 'no' can feel like a smack in the face even though there may be a very good reason for your partner's lack of interest. There are many ways to communicate interest to your partner. Some people prefer the non-verbal approach as a low-risk method of communicating desire. I have clients who place a teddy bear on each other's pillow whenever one of them is interested in sex. Another couple signals interest with a lit candle on the bedside table. Even if an uninterested partner tosses the teddy bear or blows out the candle, it's a little easier to take than a cold shoulder when you reach for your partner under the covers.

## The Set-Up

For some, morning sex is the best way to start the day. For others who are comatose until they shower and have coffee, it's about as appealing as a root canal. For low desire men, the morning may be the best time for sex because of higher testosterone levels. If you want morning sex and your partner doesn't, find out if there are certain circumstances which can make morning sex a more appealing option. Serving your partner coffee or juice in bed followed by the offer of a full body scrub in the shower might stir some interest. Or compromise with a nooner. Due to the exhaustion factor, it's a challenge for most low desire people to feel much interest in sex during the week. But maybe there are circumstances that would make it more inviting. Taking time for a hot bath or watching an erotic movie together on Wednesday night could give 'hump' day a whole new meaning.

Context is as important as timing. For some people, it's important to shower together before becoming intimate. Some people like getting it on *in* the shower, and others like getting messy with whipped cream and showering afterward. Any way you slice it, water is a wonderful medium for both cleanliness and sex play. There are those who prefer quickies and others who don't enjoy sex unless there's plenty of time for extended foreplay – and a long nap afterward. Where sex occurs can be stimulating or inhibiting. Making love on your parents' bed while they're away for the weekend could go either way, depending on your psyche. Certain smells can be a sensual turn-on or a turn-off. It's important to let your partner know to skip the garlic on date night if the scent is enough to have you sleeping in the guest room. Sounds and specific kinds of music are often arousing or at least a cover for sex noise. There's endless variety to our sexual maps, and getting to know your partner's map in greater detail is part of the adventure.

## Desire Differences

How often do you want to have sex? If you and your partner come up with the same number, congratulations! You're one of the rare couples who are perfectly matched in the desire department. For everyone else on the planet, managing the differences in desire without conflict and resentment requires good communication and a commitment to working together. Somewhere between you and your partner's ideal frequencies is probably where you're going to find the most satisfaction. But negotiating differences is more than a simple compromise. Really, what's the compromise between every day and once a month? Managing desire differences is about both partners valuing the physical side of their relationship as well as recognizing the different needs, feelings, and obstacles that each brings to their intimacy.

Dr. Pat Love, author of *Hot Monogamy* and *The Truth About Love*, is a self-confessed low desire person. In one of her workshops, she shared how little she understood what it was like to experience true sexual hunger until she received testosterone supplements as part of her research on sexuality. The boost in testosterone created a physical drive and longing for sex she'd never previously experienced. She remarked that it was like an itch needing to be scratched – and that going without sex created an actual sense of physical discomfort. It was an eye-opening experiment for Dr. Love that forever changed how she related to her higher desire partner's sexual needs.

If you're the higher desire partner, you've probably been accused of "only caring about sex". In order for your partner to understand what's going on inside your mind and body, it's helpful to explain how you experience your sexual drive and why sex is important to you. Discuss what it's like for you when there are long dry spells in your lovemaking. If your partner has little natural desire, your experience of sexuality may be foreign. It is, therefore, your responsibility to demonstrate caring in your partner's language, which probably isn't goosing them as they pour their morning coffee. If sex helps you connect to your partner, make sure they're getting that message. Then, begin stretching beyond your own frame of reference to help your partner connect to you.

If you're the lower desire partner, explain your difficulty with getting in the mood and what it's like to lack spontaneous desire. Describe the obstacles you must overcome to feel receptive and responsive to physical closeness. You've probably been accused of "never wanting to have sex". It's up to you to begin working on the physical expression of your love. If that feels like too much effort, just consider what it's like when your partner isn't doing what makes *you* feel loved. You probably expect your partner to work on meeting your needs even if it doesn't come easily to them – like listening when they don't feel like listening and expressing appreciation when silence is easier. Sex may be as important to your partner's well-being and relationship satisfaction as being heard or feeling appreciated is to your satisfaction. If your idea of foreplay is more emotional than physical, let your partner know how it is that you connect. Then translate that connection into touch.

It's important to engage in problem-solving rather than blaming. Agree to work together to make sex a priority and commit to a common goal. Get determined to make sex work for your relationship rather than against it. The more you're able to talk about how you each experience yourselves as sexual beings, the closer you'll get to understanding and meshing your sexual differences.

## You Like What??

Many couples are surprised by each other's responses to sex questionnaires even when they have been lovers for years. However, the questionnaire follow-up discussion is not the time to respond with outrage, such as, "I can't believe that for all these years you've acted like you enjoyed having your toes sucked! What else haven't you told me?" Try the questionnaire at the end of this chapter. Be prepared for surprises and open to learning new information. If there are things your partner wants you to do that you're not comfortable doing, share your feelings about that. Include anything that might make a difference in your willingness to experiment.

In a healthy relationship, both partners are willing to adapt and grow to accommodate each other's needs – in all areas. You push yourself to do things you wouldn't normally do. You go to your partner's company picnic even though you don't know anyone and would much prefer to stay home and watch a movie. You go to bed a little earlier than you'd like so that you won't be a zombie when your partner gets you up for a morning run. But then, when it comes to the sexual part of your relationship, you feel entitled to refuse any behavior that isn't already a part of your repertoire. Of course you have the right to refuse, but an unwillingness to accommodate your partner's desires often creates conflict and resentment, not to mention boredom. The intimacy in your relationship increases when both of you are willing to grow sexually. That growth also keeps your sexual life vital and satisfying.

**Fantasies**

Fantasy involves using your imagination, and can be a gold mine of material for enriching your sex life if you can stop your inner censor from spoiling all the fun. Guilt and inhibition can make it difficult to let go and experiment, even when the experimentation is confined to your own imagination. Many people have private fantasies that are never shared with a partner. Sharing your personal sex imaginings requires a great deal of trust and safety within your relationship. There is often fear of judgment from a partner – especially if the fantasy is a little kinky or bizarre – and depending on the fantasy and the partner, the fear may be justified. It's possible that your partner might feel threatened by a particular fantasy. There is always some risk involved in such intimate sharing. The risk can be reduced if you start small by revealing fantasies that are likely to be non-threatening. And if you're a high desire person, you might want to tread carefully until you're sure that your partner is comfortable with your level of sharing. It's also important to be clear about whether you have any desire to incorporate elements of the fantasy into your sexual relationship. Many couples enjoy enacting certain fantasies and find that it adds interest and intensity to their love life. Other fantasies might be strictly off-limits for enactment, but still add excitement when entertained in your mind. It's up to you to assess the safety of disclosing your private sexual visualizations. The potential rewards include increased intimacy and as much sexual variety as you can imagine.

## Specific Problems

Any sex problems you're having are probably not going to go away on their own. In fact, they're probably going to get worse unless you begin talking about them. You may think you've tried that already, but if your talking has been complaining, nagging, and arguing, then you've not yet begun a real dialogue. The dialogue begins when you're able to discuss problems without blame or criticism.

## Sharing Suggestions

I know a man who got a real jolt when his wife called the office unexpectedly and graphically described all of the things she wanted to do to him when he got home from work. He was so shocked by the call that his work day was shot, but he was shaken out of his sexual stupor and the couple had terrific sex that night. Actually it was before supper. It's important to let your partner know what they can do that enhances your interest in sex. I know of no better aphrodisiac for some women than their partners' offer to clean up the kitchen after dinner. Maybe it's feeling valued for something *other* than sex that turns you on. Clue your partner in on the romantic currency of a walk after dinner or a special night out. The important thing is to let your partner in on any secret start-ups to your sexual desire.

## Final Thoughts

In a survey of 100,000 married women, the wives' ability to talk about sex with their husbands was the strongest indicator of sexual satisfaction. And the more they talked, the happier they rated their sex lives. So, don't give up if your first attempts to talk about sex leave you feeling less like Dr. Ruth and more like Homer Simpson. If this is a new skill set for you, why would you expect to be an expert right from the start? Be prepared to be a beginner – to stumble, choke on your words, get red in the face, and possibly get a poor response from your partner. Because this is an uncomfortable proposition, it's easy to go scurrying back into your comfort zone at the first sign of trouble. Keep trying. It will get easier with practice.

It's a messy business to mesh different sexual needs and wants. It feels risky to open up to your partner, but by breaking through the barriers of fear and insecurity with your partner, you'll take your relationship to a new level of emotional intimacy. And with more intimacy comes better sex.

Jean A. Campbell

## *Sexual Response Inventory*

Next to each item, rank your enjoyment of the described activity. After you and your partner have both completed the inventory, share your responses with each other. Take note of the activities that you both enjoy. Without judgment, discuss the activities that you and your partner have ranked differently and consider possibilities for narrowing the gap in your rankings. Refrain from any pressure – this is strictly exploratory.

Rank your enjoyment on a scale of 0-5

5 Extremely Enjoyable

4 Enjoyable

3 Okay

2 Sometimes Enjoyable

1 Not Enjoyable

0 No Way, Jose

| | | | | | | |
|---|---|---|---|---|---|---|
| 1. Being seen naked | 5 | 4 | 3 | 2 | 1 | 0 |
| 2. Seeing your partner naked | 5 | 4 | 3 | 2 | 1 | 0 |
| 3. Kissing on the lips | 5 | 4 | 3 | 2 | 1 | 0 |
| 4. Deep kissing (tongues in mouths) | 5 | 4 | 3 | 2 | 1 | 0 |
| 5. Making Out (clothes on) | 5 | 4 | 3 | 2 | 1 | 0 |
| 6. Making Out (clothes off) | 5 | 4 | 3 | 2 | 1 | 0 |
| 7. Giving a non-sexual massage | 5 | 4 | 3 | 2 | 1 | 0 |
| 8. Receiving a non-sexual massage | 5 | 4 | 3 | 2 | 1 | 0 |
| 9. Kissing and sucking partner's breasts and nipples | 5 | 4 | 3 | 2 | 1 | 0 |

| | | | | | | |
|---|---|---|---|---|---|---|
| 10. Having your breasts and nipples kissed and sucked | 5 | 4 | 3 | 2 | 1 | 0 |
| 11. Stroking your partner's genitals | 5 | 4 | 3 | 2 | 1 | 0 |
| 12. Having your genitals stroked | 5 | 4 | 3 | 2 | 1 | 0 |
| 13. Stimulating partner's genitals to orgasm | 5 | 4 | 3 | 2 | 1 | 0 |
| 14. Having your genitals stimulated to orgasm | 5 | 4 | 3 | 2 | 1 | 0 |
| 15. Licking and kissing partner's genitals | 5 | 4 | 3 | 2 | 1 | 0 |
| 16. Having your genitals licked and kissed | 5 | 4 | 3 | 2 | 1 | 0 |
| 17. Bringing partner to orgasm through oral sex | 5 | 4 | 3 | 2 | 1 | 0 |
| 18. Having partner bring you to orgasm through oral sex | 5 | 4 | 3 | 2 | 1 | 0 |
| 19. Missionary-style intercourse (man on top) | 5 | 4 | 3 | 2 | 1 | 0 |
| 20. Intercourse with woman on top | 5 | 4 | 3 | 2 | 1 | 0 |
| 21. Side by side intercourse | 5 | 4 | 3 | 2 | 1 | 0 |
| 22. Doggy-style intercourse (rear-entry) | 5 | 4 | 3 | 2 | 1 | 0 |
| 23. Intercourse standing up | 5 | 4 | 3 | 2 | 1 | 0 |
| 24. Acting out fantasies | 5 | 4 | 3 | 2 | 1 | 0 |
| 25. Talking 'dirty' during sex | 5 | 4 | 3 | 2 | 1 | 0 |
| 26. Stroking partner's buttocks and anus | 5 | 4 | 3 | 2 | 1 | 0 |
| 27. Having your buttocks and anus stroked | 5 | 4 | 3 | 2 | 1 | 0 |

| | | | | | | |
|---|---|---|---|---|---|---|
| 28. Kissing your partner's buttocks and anus | 5 | 4 | 3 | 2 | 1 | 0 |
| 29. Having your buttocks and anus kissed | 5 | 4 | 3 | 2 | 1 | 0 |
| 30. Keeping eyes open during intercourse | 5 | 4 | 3 | 2 | 1 | 0 |
| 31. Using a vibrator during sex | 5 | 4 | 3 | 2 | 1 | 0 |
| 32. Using sex toys and props during sex | 5 | 4 | 3 | 2 | 1 | 0 |
| 33. Quickies – sex that lasts less than 15 min. | 5 | 4 | 3 | 2 | 1 | 0 |
| 34. Sex that lasts 15-30 min. | 5 | 4 | 3 | 2 | 1 | 0 |
| 35. Sex that lasts 30-60 min. | 5 | 4 | 3 | 2 | 1 | 0 |
| 36. Cuddling after sex | 5 | 4 | 3 | 2 | 1 | 0 |
| 37. Being tied up or restrained during sex | 5 | 4 | 3 | 2 | 1 | 0 |
| 38. Watching pornography before or during sex | 5 | 4 | 3 | 2 | 1 | 0 |
| 39. Watching partner masturbate | 5 | 4 | 3 | 2 | 1 | 0 |
| 40. Masturbating in front of partner | 5 | 4 | 3 | 2 | 1 | 0 |
| 41. Having sex in new places | 5 | 4 | 3 | 2 | 1 | 0 |
| 42. Videotaping of lovemaking | 5 | 4 | 3 | 2 | 1 | 0 |
| 43. Having sex in the shower | 5 | 4 | 3 | 2 | 1 | 0 |
| 44. Talking after sex | 5 | 4 | 3 | 2 | 1 | 0 |
| 45. Spooning after sex | 5 | 4 | 3 | 2 | 1 | 0 |

# Dirty Word Game

Here's a fun exercise that can break down some barriers and open up new possibilities for hot sex talk. With your partner, write down all of the slang terms you can think of for the following words:

| | |
|---|---|
| Penis | Vagina |
| Vulva | Breasts |
| Testicles | Clitoris |
| Intercourse | Fellatio |
| Cunnilingus | Ejaculation |
| Masturbation | |

When you've finished your lists, talk about which words are 'hot' words for you and which ones leave you cold - and why. Let your partner know if there are words you're only comfortable hearing or using when you're in the heat of passion.

Now go back to your lists and see if you can come up with your own slang for each of the terms – maybe pet names for each other's genitals or your own terms for favorite lovemaking activities.

# Chapter 9

## Rebooting Your Partner — Without Getting the Boot

Maybe you are the higher desire partner in your relationship and have picked up this book to give to your lower desire mate. Unfortunately, your 'gift' will probably be greeted with about the same degree of enthusiasm as you received when you brought home the furry handcuffs. I want to talk about how you can approach your mate in such a way that you'll get a different response than the one you've always gotten. You've probably been doing the same thing over and over – maybe with progressively greater intensity over time – hoping that something different might happen. If your current strategy for getting more action in the bedroom is nagging, complaining, exploding, or pouting, you need a new skill set.

New skills were the topic of a conversation I had not long ago with a man in my yoga class. He was very interested in the subject of my book because he'd recently initiated an attempt to recharge his sexual relationship with his wife. He and his wife had been happily married for over 30 years, but during the last half of their marriage, their love life had gradually dwindled to almost nothing. He confided that he'd recently taken a risk and brought home a book on sexual techniques. He was pleasantly surprised by his wife's positive response, but despite that promising start, he was terrified that he might do something that would put his wife's rejuvenated interest into reverse. As he shared his tentative approaches with his wife, I had the visual image of someone carefully navigating a field of land mines. It was okay for her to initiate sexual conversation, but not okay for him to initiate it. When they did begin a sexual conversation, there were certain words he couldn't use without turning her off, but he wasn't quite certain what words were prohibited. She wanted him to show sexual interest in her, but wanted a softer approach than the one he'd been using for the last 30 years. Despite their many years of marriage, my friend felt like an inexperienced newlywed trying to figure out the sexual landscape and the proper rules of engagement. He was eager and willing, however, to do anything and everything in his power to put new life into their sexual relationship. He just wanted to make sure he didn't mess things up.

If sex is MIA in your relationship or if you just want to generate more sexual interest from a generally unenthusiastic and unresponsive partner, you may wonder how to get on the fast track to success. I want to help you discover effective strategies for arousing your partner's sexual interest and desire. No matter how long it's been since you've shared a passionate kiss, felt your partner's hungry gaze, or been invited into the shower, it's not too late to revive your lover's lagging libido.

## Relationship Assessment

Before you make any move toward awakening your partner's desire, you need to first take the temperature of your relationship. Putting sex aside for a minute, use the following questions as a starting point for assessing the strength of your connection in non-sexual areas:

- How do you and your partner get along?
- Do you enjoy each other's company?
- Do you make each other laugh?
- Do you talk about something other than the next scheduled lawn care application?
- Are you kind to each other?
- Do you resolve conflicts without sarcasm, put-downs, or name-calling?
- Do you share equally in the care of the house and the children?
- Do you both feel a sense of power in the relationship?
- Are you both getting your non-sexual needs met reasonably well?
- Do you work together to create financial security?
- Do you trust each other?

You may wonder what these issues have to do with sex, but if the answer to any of the above questions is 'no', the probability of successfully rebooting your partner's sex drive is slim. Your sex life doesn't exist in a vacuum. Your bed holds the two of you *and* the sink load of dirty dishes from two days ago, the mounting credit card bills, the below-the- belt comments from last week's argument, and the silence over dinner. Until you fix the big sources of friction and distance in your relationship, you can't reasonably expect your partner to enthusiastically embrace your goal of a lusty love life. Don't trust that your answers to the above questions tell the whole story, either. Ask your partner the same questions, and if your answers differ, don't get defensive – get curious instead, and listen carefully to your partner. Determine what needs aren't being met in the relationship, and begin working harder to meet those needs.

## You Get Points for Effort

If you're feeling discouraged at this point (i.e. I didn't know I was going to have to perform miracles!), here's the good news: You don't have to create the perfect marriage before sparking your partner's interest in sex. What you must do is invest more effort into meeting their needs, and demonstrate your genuine interest in being a better partner. In the past, you may have used your partner's sexual shutdown as a justification for withholding what they wanted from you. Poor strategy. It's time to stop thinking about what your partner deserves, and start thinking about what they want. Withholding what your partner wants from you as a punishment for sexual rejection will never get you the sex that you want. Let me say that in another way to make sure you understand: If you act like a jerk (or a jerkette) when you don't get the sex you want, you're going to be jerking off a lot! It's only through building an atmosphere of safety and good will that your sex life can be revived.

## Create Safety

Safety is critical because without it, trust is impossible. Without trust, your partner will be reluctant to take the risks that are involved in being sexual. Passion involves the ability to let go and to be vulnerable. Your partner is unlikely to let go if they don't trust in your friendship and love. That's why *you* have to be the one to take the first step away from the 'withholding as punishment' cycle. Yes, I know your partner may withhold, as well – they withhold sex and you withhold whatever they need from you. But if you wait for your partner to make the first move, you give up all of your power to create change. You can continue the standoff, or you can decide to start using a strategy that has a better probability of success. A couple I saw for joint therapy was stuck in just such a standoff:

> Cindy and Carl had both been feeling victimized in their relationship for a long time, and neither felt any inclination to change unless they first got what they wanted. For Cindy, that was getting more of Carl's attention, and for Carl, it was getting more sex from Cindy. Cindy had no interest in having sex with a man who barely even talked to her – but Carl was so hurt and angry over Cindy's sexual rejection that he just shut down and turned away from her emotionally. When each was finally able to see the other's pain, a door opened for change. They agreed to have a date night once a week and began to take a 30-minute walk after dinner every evening. Cindy was thrilled to 'have her husband back' and was even able to initiate

sex for the first time in months. Feeling desired was powerful reinforcement for Carl who started making a point to ask Cindy about her day during their evening walk. In the standoff, neither Carl nor Cindy were getting their needs met. When Carl stepped out of the victim role and began paying attention to Cindy, both were able to soften their positions and start moving toward one another.

## Sexual Safety

In addition to the general safety within your relationship that grows out of caring, respect, and fair fighting, your partner needs to feel a specific sense of safety in your sexual connection, as well. Though I'm far more interested in "do's" than "don'ts", I want to throw out a few cautions in the interest of creating sexual safety:

- Don't ever make negative remarks to others about your sexual relationship with your partner. Protect your partner's privacy.
- Don't put pressure on your partner to have sex.
- Don't push your partner to do sexual things that make them uncomfortable.
- Don't criticize your partner with sexual put-downs – ever, ever, ever.
- Don't negatively critique your partner's body – even slightly. I can assure you that your partner is already self-conscious about their physical imperfections.
- Don't dwell on the frustrations or failures of the past.

These guidelines protect the trust and vulnerability of your partner. Avoiding criticism and pressure creates not only safety, but a positive and healthy sexual dynamic, as well.

## Re-romanticize

There's one more step you should take before approaching your partner about your sex life. Work on building more romance into your relationship – without expecting a sexual 'reward'. Small acts of love and caring are significant in restoring a sense of connection. Flowers and candlelit dinners are wonderful, but don't save all of your romance for the grand gestures. Putting more romance into your daily life with your partner will actually have a bigger impact. Your courtship was probably characterized by cards, love notes, small gifts, thoughtful gestures, and routine courtesies. If these acts have disappeared from your relationship, it's time to bring them back. Increase affectionate touch (and at this stage, grabbing your partner's genitals does not count as affectionate touch). A hug, a kiss on the back of the neck, a squeeze of a shoulder, and a caress on the face all communicate caring and tenderness to your mate. Hold hands when you're walking together, get out of your favorite chair and have couch-time with your partner while watching TV, do an impromptu dance around the kitchen when a favorite oldie comes on the radio, give your partner a foot massage, or rub your partner's shoulders when they're hunched over a computer keyboard. There's no shortage of opportunities for touch.

Whether it's a touch, a compliment, a gift, or a simple phone call to say 'I love you', make it a point to do something on a daily basis that injects positive energy into your relationship. Engage in conversation about something other than the noises coming from your ancient water heater. Stop assuming that you know everything there is to know about your partner, and revive the curiosity you felt in the beginning of your relationship. In many ways, your lover is still a mystery who is always evolving. Ray's story illustrates this point:

> Ray had been married to Helen for 23 years and assumed he knew her inside and out. However, he got a wakeup call one night when they had some friends over. Everyone was talking about the weather turning colder, and Ray casually mentioned how much Helen hated the winter season. Helen very pointedly corrected him, saying that she *had* hated winter at one time but had come to a real appreciation and enjoyment of all the seasons. It was a perspective she had shared with Ray but apparently hadn't registered with him. Ray was reminded of the need to keep listening and learning as a way of loving his life partner.

## Have the 'Talk'

After getting your relationship on more solid ground and creating an atmosphere of safety and romance, it's time to talk to your partner about why you feel the sexual part of your relationship is important. Pick a time and a place when you're both relaxed and feeling connected. Share what you get from your lovemaking and what rewards you anticipate for both of you if there is an improvement in your sex life. Avoid blaming your partner for whatever problems there have been in your sexual relationship, and don't attempt to 'guilt' your partner into jumping on the rebooting bandwagon. Stay positively focused.

Together, recall the early times in your relationship and what was special about your sex life. Reminisce about memorable sexual experiences. Talk about the most unusual places you've had sex. Get out your old photo albums and look at pictures from your courtship or your honeymoon. Think about how much time you devoted to being together and the careful planning that went into arranging fun outings. Remember and share what attracted you to one another and what fueled your sexual chemistry.

In the years following your intoxicating beginnings, it's not always easy to stay closely connected to your partner. If your relationship has slowly slipped down on your list of priorities, both of you have contributed to this decline. Apologize for the ways in which you've neglected your mate and allowed distance to creep into the relationship. Let your partner know that you regret any negativity or pressure you've been responsible for in your sexual relationship, as well. Invite your partner to talk about changes they've experienced in their sexuality and obstacles they face in maintaining intimacy. Acknowledge the differences that exist between your levels of sexual desire without assigning positive or negative value to those differences.

If your partner indicates a willingness to work on improving your sex life, ask how you can make that easier. Let them know you no longer want to pressure for sex, but you do want to learn how to stimulate their sexual interest. Find out how they like to be approached when you're interested in sex or whether they need a period of time in which you allow them to be the sole initiator of sexual activity.

Turning over the responsibility for initiating sex to the lower desire partner is often helpful in disrupting the negative cycle of pressure and resistance which may have come to characterize your attempts to initiate sex. If your partner wants you to continue initiating, ask them to identify the conditions and times of day when you are most likely to get a 'yes'. Introduce the concept of scaling in which part of your sexual approach is to ask your partner to rate their interest in sex on a scale from 1 to 10. Decide together how to interpret the numbers.

For example:
- 1-2 Absolutely not. I'm tired, sick, fed up, etc. It would take a major miracle and a week at a resort to get me in the mood.
- 3-4 Not feeling any interest, but sex is not completely out of the question.
- 5-6 Not exactly raring to go, but I could be enticed with the right moves.
- 7-8 I'm interested – it wouldn't take much to activate my desire.
- 9-10 This is as good as it gets – where are the handcuffs?

Using this scale, a 1 or 2 means drop it immediately – another word and your reboot is in jeopardy. Anything between a 3 and a 6 means you're still in the game, but you want to tread carefully. This would be the time to ask your partner what you could do to move them from say, a 5 to a 7. And don't assume that the response will be something like, "Go get into your thong" or "Pop in the sex video", either. The reply may be more along the lines of, "Clean up the kitchen" or "Let the dogs out".

In approaching your partner or in talking about sex, it's important to use words your partner finds comfortable. Find out if there are off-putting words that you need to avoid and whether your partner's comfort with certain sexual language changes depending upon the context. My yoga friend was shocked to discover that his wife actually liked being called a 'slut' when they were having sex. She found that it turned her on – but only after she'd gotten warmed up a little. That's important information. My friend would have hell to pay if he called his wife a slut in any other context.

I know one couple who made up their own game for getting more comfortable with using sexual words. They each made up a stack of cards with names of body parts or sexual acts printed on each one. Whoever lost each hand of their favorite card game had to draw a card from their partner's stack and say aloud whatever was printed on the card. Be creative in coining your own terms for each other's genitalia and sexual acts, but always be willing to accommodate your partner's preferred language.

## Maximize Interest

In addition to language preferences, find out how you can play to your partner's desire through how you present yourself. Ask how they like to see you dress. You may be surprised by their answers. Find out what clothes or particular outfits your partner finds sexy and stimulating. Ask what kind of underwear they like to see you in. Some women prefer boxers over briefs on their man and silk over cotton. It's assumed that men are turned on by the sight of their lover in a thong and a lacy bra, but I know some men who find nothing more enticing than white cotton panties and a plain white bra. Some accommodation to your partner's clothing preferences – at least when you're in the mood for love – may help your partner to get turned on.

Don't neglect the other senses when attempting to maximize your partner's interest. Do they like you clean-shaven or is the rough feel of a two-day stubble their idea of a turn-on? Do they prefer that you be freshly showered or enjoy your natural scent? Is there a mouthwash that makes your kisses more desirable? (Hint: Cinnamon has been proven to be a sexual stimulant for men. Baby powder has the same effect on women, but I wouldn't recommend gargling with it.) Does your partner like you to wear cologne? Any particular one? Is it important to your partner that you take special care of your fingernails and toenails? Does your partner like you to wear makeup or does he prefer the natural look? How does your partner like you to wear your hair? Try dressing and grooming to your partner's liking for an entire weekend instead of skipping showers and grubbing around in your faded t-shirt and cut-offs. Stop saving your hottest looks for the office.

Once you've discovered how to be a desirable partner, find out what settings your lover prefers for intimacy. Do they like music? Candlelight? A romp in the woods? How much privacy do they need? Are they extremely sensitive to the possibility of being overheard during lovemaking? Do they enjoy novelty, or do they need the comfort and familiarity of their bed in order to relax? Do they need the room to be a certain temperature? Are clean sheets more inviting? Paying attention to the setting for sex can enhance your partner's relaxation and receptivity to sexual encounters.

**Green Light!**

You're finally down to the nitty-gritty of getting it on. When your partner's desire is out of the deep freeze, and you've been given the green light to proceed, your reboot mission can now advance to the exploration of erogenous zones and preferred sexual practices. It's helpful to begin by reviving the lost art of making out – without any expectation of it leading to intercourse. Drive to a secluded spot in a park or just get cozy on the living room couch. Take each step slowly, spending a lot of time on kissing before doing any other touching. Let the passion build gradually. Take your cues from your partner in moving to more intimate kinds of contact. Depending upon your partner's response, be willing to have multiple make-out sessions without them culminating in intercourse. Let your partner know in advance that you don't have any specific sexual expectations.

When you and your partner are ready for the whole smorgasbord of sexual activity, approach this feast as a novice. You may have made love with your partner hundreds of times, but you will reap immeasurable rewards if you assume the role of a student in learning your partner's sexual responses. Your job is to be a scout of this familiar sexual terrain, and be open to new discoveries about your partner. As you explore, encourage your partner to share any discomfort that surfaces. Discomfort includes physical discomfort, as well as anything that creates uneasiness, anxiety, anger, pressure, guilt, or shame. Ask your partner to acknowledge their discomfort immediately with a non-verbal signal or a simple statement, and then give you a suggestion for how to eliminate the discomfort. Don't take their discomfort personally or interpret it as criticism – and don't try to 'talk them out of it'. Listen carefully to the problem, and work together toward a solution. In addition to encouraging your partner to share any discomfort, it's equally important to receive positive feedback when something feels right. Positive reinforcement is a powerful tool in teaching you exactly how to give pleasure.

## Reinforce Positive Changes

Be patient with your partner, and continue to let them know how much it means to you that they are willing to make your sexual relationship a higher priority. Remember that if your partner doesn't experience spontaneous feelings of desire, it's easy for them to let the sexual side of your relationship slide. Unlike you, your lower desire partner has to be very intentional about creating space and energy for sex to occur. That requires a major commitment. If your partner returns to old patterns of avoiding or neglecting your sexual relationship, refrain from matching their relapse with one of your own. *Do not* sabotage their efforts to change by becoming critical, angry, or resigned ("I knew this wouldn't last"). Approach your partner gently, and let them know you've missed the physical intimacy in your relationship. Find out what's been going on with them that may have interfered with their availability. Ask if there's anything you can do to help the two of you get back on track. Focus on *being* the loving partner you want to have.

## Final Thoughts

If your ideal sexual frequency is once a day and your partner finds weekly sex a stretch, it's unlikely that even your best efforts at being a loving mate are going to get you daily sex.

Successful relationships involve an acceptance of differences and a willingness to accommodate. Chances are, as you improve the quality of your sexual relationship, the quantity will become less important. Like a dieter who obsesses over chocolate following weeks of chocolate deprivation, those who have been on a forced sex diet tend to obsess over sex. When your partner's interest is rekindled and you reclaim some of the sexual synergy you once had with each other, your sense of deprivation will fade. You may then be surprised to find that sex once or twice a week is more than satisfying.

# *Exercise*

Are you being the most loving partner you can be? Are there things you need to do differently if you want a more interested sex partner? Take a look at the following list, and do an honest appraisal of yourself as a partner.

T  F  I make a real effort to get along with my partner

T  F  I frequently laugh with my partner

T  F  I have good conversations with my partner – both listening and sharing

T  F  I carry my share of responsibility for the house and the family

T  F  I am able to discuss differences without yelling, sarcasm, or put-downs

T  F  My partner can count on me to do what I say I'm going to do

T  F  I am financially responsible

T  F  I invite my partner's participation in decision-making

T  F  I make a real effort not to pout or withdraw when my partner turns down sex

T  F  I am caring, kind, and respectful toward my partner

T  F  I keep the sex life with my partner private

T  F  I don't pressure my partner to have sex or to do sexual things they don't want to do

T  F  I refrain from sexual put-downs and negative comments about my partner's body

T  F  I put regular effort into being romantic and affectionate with my partner

T  F  I avoid blame and guilt when I talk to my partner about our sex life

T  F  I take responsibility for my contribution to the problems in our relationship

T  F  I accept my partner's differences without labeling them as bad or wrong

T  F  I ask my partner what I can do to increase their sexual interest

T  F  I'm open to compromise and accommodation in our sexual relationship

T  F  I'm sensitive to the language my partner finds comfortable for talking about sex

T  F  I make an effort to look, smell, and feel good for my partner

T  F  I try to create an atmosphere for sex that is pleasing to my partner

T  F  I kiss and touch my partner without always expecting it will lead to intercourse

T  F  I am open to learning more about my partner's sexual responses and preferences

T  F  I am not defensive when my partner shares discomfort with certain sexual touch

T  F  I express appreciation for my partner's willingness to work on our sexual relationship

For any statements that you circled as false, try writing down a commitment for change that will help spark your partner's sexual interest.

I will _____

_____

_____

_____

I will _____

_____

_____

_____

I will _____

_____

_____

_____

I will _____

_____

_____

_____

# Chapter 10

## Tricks of the Trade: Tips for Keeping Yourself Turned On

In previous chapters, I discussed the importance of physical and emotional health in the flow of sexual energy as well as the relationship issues which can sideline even the healthiest of libidos. Once you've addressed negative programming, gotten your life in balance, and put your relationship on solid ground, you may still find it a challenge to keep your libido in full gear. Keeping your sex life rich and rewarding involves a commitment to make sex a priority – both individually and as a couple. That commitment entails a clear intention to increase awareness of your sexuality.

### Decide to Be Sexy

Now that you know why it's a mistake to stash your sexuality in the back of the closet with the old tuxedo and prom dresses, you can start putting more energy into being sexy – not just for your partner, but for yourself. Make a decision to start acting more sexual. Indulge in occasional sexual thoughts throughout the day, and don't miss an opportunity to see, hear, smell, taste, and feel the richness of the universe around you. Dress a little differently, and notice how clothes feel against your skin. Tune into your erogenous zones, and increase your sensitivity to touch. Become more affectionate with your partner, and begin flirting and teasing again. Playing the seducer or the seductress will not only build your partner's interest, but your own as well.

> Karen, a 56-year-old client, wanted to get back the sexual relationship she'd once enjoyed with her husband, Chris. Since going through menopause, she'd lost all interest in sex and found one excuse after another to avoid it. The lack of intimacy was taking a toll on the marriage, and Karen felt guilty about her role in it. She didn't think she could make herself feel something she didn't feel, but decided to take a stab at it by ditching her dingy white undies for colorful matching lingerie. "Chris had always wanted me to wear sexy underwear, but I thought it was an unnecessary expense. When I finally treated myself to a shopping spree at Victoria's Secret, I was surprised that I actually felt kind of sexy. I hadn't felt anything even close to that for a long time. I really was only doing it for Chris, but somehow, just feeling a little sexier has changed things for both of us. I'll probably never want sex as much as Chris, but it's stopped feeling like a chore."

## Schedule Time for Sex

Don't get sucked into the romantic myth that the only good sex is spontaneous sex. 'Doing it' actually makes you want to do it more, so it's important to be intentional about keeping it on the schedule. If you wait until both you and your partner are spontaneously turned on, you may be waiting a very long time. Making sex dates with your partner is a way of saying that you both value the sexual part of your relationship and aren't willing to leave it to chance. You schedule everything else in your life - why shouldn't sex be just as important as your 7:00 kickboxing class?

Lisa and Jim have regular 'sex appointments':

> "Our sex life improved 100% after we started setting aside special times for sex. It gives us both time to get in the mood, and neither one of us has to worry about being turned down. We each shower first - sometimes together - and then put on some music and light a few candles. Sometimes we go out first, like to dinner at a nice restaurant, and begin building up to sex by flirting and touching one another under the table. We still have our quickies and that comfortable, routine kind of sex that married couples fall into, but our 'appointments' keep some excitement in our sex life."

Far from being unromantic, setting aside special time for sex gives you the opportunity to charge up your sexual battery. Just because sex is on the calendar doesn't mean it has the same routine status as your dental appointment. On the scheduled date, start the day by leaving a steamy note beside your partner's coffee cup. Later send a suggestive email from work. Expressing your anticipation can keep your scheduled time together hot *and* romantic.

## Stimulate Your Sexual Imagination

Keep a good supply of erotic literature, sexy movies, and 'dirty' magazines around to help generate interest when there's little or no spontaneous desire. You can stimulate yourself with any of this material before even approaching your partner, or together you can watch a movie or read some erotic passages aloud. Sex shops – or sex boutiques as the more fashionable ones are called – are gradually popping up on the suburban landscape, no longer confined to the seamy side of town. If there's one in your area, go browsing and check out the vibrators, lotions and sex toys that are available. Even if you don't buy anything, you might find your interest getting sparked.

Lisa and Jim started out one of their sex appointments with a field trip to a sex boutique:

> "We couldn't believe how many sex toys are out there – everything from a whole wall of vibrators and dildos to racks of dress-up outfits. Lisa picked out a French maid uniform that was perfect for acting out one of my fantasies. It was a little pricey – but worth every penny."

## Make a Love Nest

Before you go to bed tonight, take an inventory of your bedroom. Is there a treadmill you're using as a clothes rack? Are there bills that haven't yet been filed and stacks of magazines you'll never have time to read? When your bedroom is cluttered and disorganized, it's hardly a relaxing and sensual environment for lovemaking. Try clearing out the extraneous distractions, and aim for simplicity and serenity. Make sure the room is a pleasing color and has soft lighting available. Invest in the best quality cotton sheets you can find (satin is sexy but too slippery for traction), and have plenty of soft, inviting pillows on the bed. Keep lotions and tissues next to the bed, as well as some erotica and whatever sex toys you and your partner enjoy. Place scented candles around the room, and have a stereo or CD player available along with your favorite music for lovemaking. Make sure the temperature in the room is comfortable, as well (a ceiling fan is nice for keeping things from getting too overheated). Keep the bedroom a television and computer-free zone. Lying next to someone who's clicking away on their laptop or dozing off while watching Letterman is not conducive to lovemaking or good sleep. Feel free to lock the door to your couple retreat, and don't answer the phone unless the call is from the hospital or the police station. Creating your own love nest increases the odds that you'll use it more often for making love.

**Explore Touch**

When you've been doing something for 20, 30, 40 years or more, it's easy to assume that you know all there is to know about it. That's the attitude many people have toward sex – and that I had about driving. Last year, I got a speeding ticket and ended up in traffic school to avoid having points added to my license. I was more than a little irritated and assumed I'd be sitting through several hours of boring drivel. I was surprised to find that I actually learned a few things – besides the penalty for disregarding the speed limit. There may only be a finite amount to learn about driving, but sexual learning is virtually inexhaustible – not only because there's a wealth of sexual information available, but because your own sexuality and that of your partner is constantly changing. It's important to learn what pleases your partner sexually and to teach your partner what pleases you. Take your newly developed skill in sex talk and couple it with exploratory contact. Ask your partner to alternate being the giver and then the receiver of touch. When you're in the receiving role, your job is to give very specific feedback to your partner about the kind of touch you want. It's best to begin this exercise by touching the scalp and then moving very slowly down the entire body and the extremities, saving the breasts and the genitals for last. As the giver of touch, your job is to listen very carefully to your partner's feedback and adjust your touch to meet their needs. Recognizing that there is always something new to learn and remaining open to new input allows your sexuality to grow and evolve. Maintaining a sexual dialogue with your partner ensures that you stay on the path of sexual learning.

## Keep It Fresh

I often hear clients describe the predictable and uninspired routine that has come to characterize virtually every sexual encounter with their partner, and I can understand why it might be difficult to get turned on. As one client complained to me, "When he wants sex, he reaches for my breasts. After about 2 minutes of kneading my breasts, he moves his hand down between my legs and starts stroking my clitoris. After about 2-3 minutes of that, he gets on top of me and a minute later, we're done." This is not to say that predictability is all bad. We often find comfort in the familiar, especially when we're tired and don't really want swinging-from-the-chandeliers sex. However, too much routine in your sexual relationship creates the identical boredom you may feel with the monotony of your everyday life. It's no wonder affairs are so exciting – they offer novelty, variety, and intensity – but you don't have to risk the devastation of an affair in order to have a more interesting sex life.

You can give your relationship more zing and make it more affair-proof by engineering some of that excitement in your sex life with your partner. One of the big factors in eroticism is unpredictability. Think about your very earliest sexual encounters with your partner. One of the powerful turn-ons was not knowing what was coming next or how far things were going to go. After settling in with your partner, a lot of that mystery disappears. That doesn't mean there can't still be an element of surprise in your lovemaking. Being unpredictable keeps the passion alive long after the honeymoon is over – and the unexpected doesn't have to be big or elaborate.

In addition to new sex toys, hot lingerie, and shared fantasies, you can experiment with new positions or new sexual behaviors to spice up your lovemaking. Simply introducing some variety in how you initiate sex can help. Maybe the man who went straight for his wife's breasts as his start-up standby could change the routine by first nibbling on her earlobe or stroking her hair. Varying the amount of time devoted to lovemaking can also provide a welcome change to the sexual routine. Everything from a quickie to an evening-long sexual date can be satisfying depending upon the circumstances and the time available. There are plenty of books available on-line and in your local bookstore illustrating sexual techniques that your imagination alone may not generate. Every couple could benefit from a few of these books on their shelf.

One of the great things about introducing novelty into your sex life is that the excitement it generates lasts far beyond the initial encounter. Because our brains work by association, that one fantastic sexual adventure where your wrists were tied to the bed posts with silk scarves infuses new energy into your sex life for months – or even years – to come. So luckily, you don't have to be creative and adventurous every single time you make love. You can revisit past adventures, and allow your memories to stir your passion.

Over the years, my husband and I have collected many memories that we use to pull ourselves out of the sexual doldrums. One of our favorites is from our 15th anniversary vacation in Hawaii. Before leaving for the trip, I secretly bought a long, black wig and packed it alongside a new dress with a plunging neck line. What woman hasn't wanted to look like Cher at least once in her life? Though it required careful planning, I decided that a snorkeling trip we had scheduled would give me a chance to do my changing act. Following snorkeling, looking more than a little worse for the wear, I ducked into the outfitter's changing room and began my transformation. I quickly changed into the dress and heels, put on my makeup and wig, and sauntered out to meet my husband. Waiting in our rented convertible, he looked at me first without recognition and then did a double-take. He continued staring at me during dinner with a look I hadn't felt for a very long time. Now I'm not sure what kind of sex Cher has, but our evening culminated in a liaison that I'd venture to say was pretty atypical for an old married couple – a one-night stand with a new version of me that not only didn't jeopardize our relationship but brought it new excitement and vitality. Does that sound like a lot of trouble? Really just some forethought and the kind of focus that's much easier to achieve while on vacation.

## Take a Vacation

The luxury of time and freedom from the demands of everyday life creates the perfect opportunity for you to reconnect with your partner. Couple vacations are critical for renewing a sense of partnership and rediscovering the passionate side of your love – and maybe even finding a new way of introducing yourself to your partner. Plus, everyone knows that hotel sex, even when you're *not* on vacation, is hotter and more creative than most people manage on a day-to-day basis at home. Whether it's the anonymity, the absence of a to-do list, or the centrality of the bed, hotel rooms should be fully exploited for adventurous sex.

## Take a Mini-Vacation

Most people can manage only one or two vacations a year, *if* they're lucky. A strategy for reconnecting with your partner that you may find more accessible is the scheduling of mini-vacations. Mini-vacations can take place without ever packing a suitcase. You and your partner could decide to play hooky from work and spend the day doing something you both enjoy. Or you could take a Sunday and declare it a stay-in-bed day – a day when you chuck all your normal chores, errands, and responsibilities, take the phone off the hook, and make love, nap, and feed each other grapes and cheese. If it's just too difficult for you to ignore all the things screaming to get done when you stay in the house, or if you have children at home, then take a 24 or 48 hour getaway to a nearby hotel. When my husband and I were struggling with the demands of a stepfamily and three moody, mouthy teenagers, we periodically took off to one of several cities within a 100 mile radius and spent 24 hours rediscovering the love that had spawned our wild journey together. We returned home to the same stresses and the same insanity, but were re-energized and filled up enough to commit to another round.

## Change the Setting

Any change of setting that alters the context for sex can make sexual encounters fresher and more stimulating. Even getting it on in different rooms of your house introduces some needed variety. For those of you who are adventurous, try finding secluded places in the great outdoors. My husband and I have enjoyed making love in the woods, sand dunes, meadows, lakes, streams, and oceans. Water always adds an interesting element.

## Make Sex a Gift

Never 'submit' to sex. With submission, your partner gets nothing but a physical release, and you get nothing but another heaping dose of resentment. However, if your partner is interested in sex and you're not, you can make the decision to freely give of yourself sexually to your partner. As long as one-sided sex doesn't become the norm, and as long as you can give without resentment, there's nothing wrong with satisfying your partner's sexual need in a loving manner without seeking your own sexual gratification. It might be a good time to offer a quickie or oral sex or a 'hand job'. When given with a loving spirit, there's probably no more meaningful gift you could give to your partner. It's also an investment in the relationship.

## Stay Tuned Into Your Partner's Senses

By fully engaging all of your senses, you stay tuned into your own sexuality. Through careful attention to the senses of your partner, you imprint yourself firmly in their consciousness. During your courting days, you undoubtedly went to great lengths to look, sound, feel, smell, and taste good to your partner. You worked hard to accent your sexual desirability. If you've started shlepping around the house every weekend in a sloppy sweat suit and have declared Saturday and Sunday to be hygiene-free days, you're not as likely to feel sexy or send out any sexy vibes. To bring back some of the heightened sexual interest of your dating days, begin using your senses to rev up your sex appeal.

> **Sight**: Take care of your appearance. Don't forsake all grooming tasks on the weekend, and, at least occasionally, wear something comfortable but stylish when you're hanging out at home. Display pictures of you and your partner embracing. Look deeply into your partner's eyes. Keep your eyes open while you're

making love. Take time to visually appreciate your partner's body.

**Hearing**: Be more intentional about creating soothing sounds in your home environment. Turn off the drone of the TV when no one is watching it, and replace it with your favorite music. Practice talking with a pleasing tone. If you play a musical instrument, play it for your partner. Unless you're tone deaf, sing harmony with your partner on a favorite song. Whisper romantic words or hot sex talk in your lover's ear.

**Touch**: Touch is the language of lovers, so rediscover the joys of touching your partner, both in and out of the bedroom. Touch can be playful, affectionate, passionate, relaxing, nurturing, and so much more. Practice communicating different moods and feelings to your partner strictly through touch. Maximize skin-to-skin contact by sleeping in the nude.

**Smell**: Make sure your breath is fresh and your body odor attracts rather than repels your lover. Wear the cologne your partner likes best. Create tantalizing aromas in the kitchen, and place flowers in the bedroom. The sense of smell is an important part of our sexuality. Find out what smells serve as an aphrodisiac for you and for your partner.

**Taste**: Your lips, mouth, and tongue are exquisitely tuned to give and receive pleasure with your lover. Licking, sucking, and nibbling can provide an endless variety of sexual delight. Eating is also a sensuous and pleasurable experience. Try feeding your partner and allow them to feed you. Incorporate new tastes into your lovemaking through flavored lubricants or creative use of peanut butter, whipped cream, honey, or assorted ice cream toppings.

## Indulge in Fantasy

Sexual interest begins in your mind. If your brain doesn't happen to be churning out highly sexualized thoughts and images, you can nudge it in that direction with your own sexual imaginings. If you don't have any spontaneous fantasies of your own, then borrow someone else's. Replay in your mind a hot scene from a movie like 9 ½ Weeks, recall a highly erotic scenario from a romance novel, or imagine sexual endings to everyday experiences like the UPS guy who delivers more than one kind of package, the 21-year-old babysitter who ravages you when you're taking her home, or the lonely repairman who fixes your libido after fixing your furnace. Your fantasies are exempt from your normal code of ethics, and the variations are limited only by your imagination. Approximately 85 percent of people engage in fantasy, both as a prelude to sex, as well as during sex. Men's fantasy lives are filled with visual images and a focus on the physical, whereas women's fantasies are built more around a story. Men often think about things they've actually experienced, while women are likely to fantasize about things they've never done. Just remember that having a fantasy doesn't mean you want to enact it in real life, and fantasizing forbidden activities doesn't make you a pervert.

Fantasizing allows your brain to block out distractions while increasing your desire. The following are just a few of the top male and female fantasies:

- Sex with a man or woman other than your partner
- Threesomes
- Sex with a stranger
- Seducing a virgin
- Being 'forced' to have sex
- Watching other people have sex

**Play**

Recapture the ability to play with your partner. If you can't be playmates, you're probably going to struggle with being good sex mates. Play board games, have water gun fights, take turns making up stories about strangers, go to a playground, jump together on a trampoline, do the hustle, put the soles of your feet together and bicycle, roll down a grassy hill, or go sledding. Try a few of the aforementioned activities naked. Do anything that's playful, energizing, and makes you laugh, and then incorporate some of your play into your sex life. Play strip poker or sexual charades. I know one couple who sometimes likes to play red light, green light when they're making love. 'Mother May I' might be another interesting game. Acting out fantasies can be a form of play. Playing lowers your inhibitions, activates the pleasure centers in your brain, and increases your connection with your partner. How could it not improve your sex life?

## Make Love – All Day Long

Try expanding the meaning of 'making love' to include all of the loving behaviors that you and your partner do for each other, like rubbing tired shoulders, scraping the ice off a windshield, planning an overnight getaway, or baking chocolate chip cookies. If you think more about how to make love to your partner in the non-sexual realm, you'll probably have more lovemaking of the traditional variety. When couples don't take each other for granted and are able to maintain a caring relationship, the sex flows naturally as a celebration of that caring connection. Love can be as much about *making* the bed as about making love *in* the bed.

## Get Excited

Lastly, if you want to stay passionately engaged with your partner, stay passionately engaged with life. If you're just putting time in on your job and have become cynical and jaded with politics, if you've lost a sense of meaning and purpose in life, or if you find yourself frequently bored, your sex life doesn't stand a chance. Don't expect that great sex is going to turn your life around. You'll only discover great sex after you've claimed the power to make your life what you want it to be. It's curiosity, openness, and the ability to be amazed that feeds passion, and it's feeling and caring deeply that allows you to hold up your end of a relationship. So, get off of the couch, start moving, sign up to save baby seals, make a difference in your workplace, go scuba diving, be kind to the person working the drive-thru, notice the sunset on your way home, and plan a night out on the town with your lover. Being fully alive is the only way to go – and the only route to an exciting and fulfilling sex life.

## Final Thoughts

Tolstoy once said, "Boredom is the desire for desire". You have the potential to create desire and banish boredom from your life and your relationship. The most potent aphrodisiac you have available to you doesn't come in pills, herbs, or injections. It's not dependent upon youth, and it doesn't cost a thing. It can bring someone back to life that has felt sexually dead for a long, long time, and it's probably the single biggest cause of affairs. What is this powerful and magical agent? It's an energized person who's interested in *you*. It's someone who looks at you and really sees you, who listens and actually laughs at your jokes, and who thinks you're intelligent, attractive, and sexy. Nothing fires up your sexual engine faster than that kind of focused, caring attention. Now think about the last time you gave that kind of attention to your partner, or the last time they gave it to you. Being a loving and emotionally available partner is vital in keeping your lover turned on. Keeping yourself turned on involves staying in balance, staying engaged in life, and staying aware of your sexuality.

I hope you'll make the commitment to awaken (or re-awaken)

the power that resides in your sexuality. Remember the slogan, "Make love, not war!"? By taking your sexuality out of hibernation mode, the benefits spread from you to your partner, and then into the world. Just imagine a world full of lovers, a world fueled by the energy and passion of sexuality untainted by shame, repression, and discomfort. Imagine the possibilities...

# *Exercise*

Which of the following suggestions would help spark your sexual interest? Pick a few of the ideas that appeal to you and make a specific plan for putting those ideas into action.

1.  Decide to be sexy

How:_____

_____

When:_____

_____

2.  Schedule time for sex

How:_____

_____

When:_____

_____

3.  Stimulate your sexual imagination

How:_____

_____

When:_____

_____

4.  Make a love nest

How:_____

_____

When:_____

_____

5.  Explore touch

How:_____

_____

When:_____

_____

6.  Keep it fresh

How:_____

_____

When:_____

_____

7.  Take a vacation

How:_____

_____

When:_____

_____

8.  Take a mini-vacation

How:_____

_____

When:_____

_____

9.  Change the setting

How:_____

_____

When:_____

_____

10. Make sex a gift

How:_____

_____

When:_____

_____

11. Stay tuned into your senses and those of your partner

**Sight**

How:_____

_____

When:_____

_____

**Hearing**

How:_____

_____

When:_____

_____

**Touch**

How:_____

_____

When:_____

_____

**Smell**

How:_____

_____

When:_____

_____

**Taste**

How:_____

_____

When:_____

_____

12. Develop your fantasy life
How:_____

_____

When:_____

_____

13. Recapture the ability to play
How:_____

_____

When:_____

_____

14. Get excited about life
How:_____

_____

When:_____

_____

# References

Amen, Daniel G. *Sex on the Brain.* New York: Harmony Books, 2007.

Bakos, Susan Crain. *Still Sexy.* New York: St. Martin's Press, 1999.

Berman, Laura. *Real Sex for Real Women.* New York: DK, 2008.

Berman, Laura. *The Passion Prescription.* New York: Hyperion, 2005.

Brown, Douglas. *Just Do It.* New York: Crown Publishers, 2008.

Cervenka, Kathleen. *In the Mood, Again.* Oakland: New Harbinger Publications, 2003.

Cox, Tracey. *Superhotsex.* New York: DK, 2006.

Diamond, Jed. *Male Menopause.* Naperville, IL: SourceBooks, 1998.

Goldstein, Andrew, and Brandon, Marianne. *Reclaiming Desire.* U.S.: Rodale, Inc., 2004.

Green, Shelley, and Flemons, Douglas. *Quickies.* New York: W.W. Norton & Co., 2004.

Hall, Kathryn. *Reclaiming Your Sexual Self.* Hoboken: John Wiley & Sons, Inc., 2004.

Heiman, Julia, and Lopiccolo, Joseph. *Becoming Orgasmic.* New York: Prentice Hall Press, 1988.

Hollander, Rene, Hornberger, Francine, and Levin, Michael. *Sex That (Still) Sizzles.* New York: Alpha Books, 2003.

Joannides, Paul. *Guide To Getting It On!* Saline, MI: McNaughton & Gunn, 2001.

Love, Patrica, and Robinson, Jo. *Hot Monogamy.* New York: Plume/Penguin, 1995.

Love, Pat. *The Truth About Love.* New York: Simon & Schuster, 2001.

McCarthy, Barry, and McCarthy, Emily. *Rekindling Desire.* New York: Brunner-Routledge, 2003.

Moore, Thomas. *Dark Nights of the Soul.* New York: Gotham Books, 2004.

Oates, Joyce Carol. *Black Water.* New York: The Penguin Group, 1993.

Parker, William H. M.D. and Parker, Rachel L. *A Gynecologists's Second Opinion.* New York: The Penguin Group, 1996.

Pearsall, Paul. *Super Marital Sex.* New York: Doubleday, 1987.

Roach, Mary. *Bonk.* New York: W.W. Norton & Co., 2008.

Sudo, Philip Toshio. *Zen Sex.* New York: Harper Collins Publishers, Inc., 2000.

Tokunaga, Adam. *Slow Sex Secrets.* New York: Vertical, Inc., 2008.

Wartik, Nancy. Whither Desire? *AARP,* November/December, 2007.

Weiner Davis, Michelle. *The Sex-Starved Marriage.* New York: Simon & Schuster, 2003.

Womack, William M., and Stauss, Fred. *The Marriage Bed.* Oakland: New Harbinger Publications, 1991.

Made in the USA
Lexington, KY
07 June 2011